Powerhouse Cancer Secrets

Avoiding Cancer, Colds,
the Flu, and More

~

Research, Remedies, and

Healthy Recipes

M. D. Kennedy

Medical Disclaimer

The information in this book is not intended or implied to be a substitute for professional medical advice, diagnosis, or treatment. All content is for general information only. The information in this book is provided without any representation or guarantees, express or implied. The author does not assume any risk for your use of the material found in this book. If you have any specific questions about any medical matter, you should consult your doctor or professional healthcare provider. If you are pregnant, nursing, or on any medication, please consult your healthcare provider before using any information in this book.

Also, do not give honey to children younger than the age of one. It could lead to infant botulism, a rare but potentially fatal illness.

Information is shared so others may become better educated on alternative and supplemental forms of treatment to heal from such a debilitating disease as cancer.

Acknowledgments

In my one-and-a-half years of research, I have found countless stories of healing and hope. Thanks to all of those who have shared their stories of success online. It gives us hope when we feel like we can do something to make a difference in our own lives and the lives of others.

Special thanks to:

My Trusty Editor and
Alex Du Toit, www.EarthieMama.com
Master Tonic and Ginger Ale recipes reprinted with permission

Dedication

Dedicated to my mother and aunt
and all of those who have
been affected by cancer.

May there be no more.

Genesis 1:29

And God said, Behold I have given you every herb bearing seed, which is
upon the face of all the earth, and every tree, which is the fruit of the tree
yielding seed; to you it shall be for meat.

Editor's note: Years ago, they ate the whole apple, seeds and all.

An apple a day on going to bed,
and you'll keep the doctor from earning his bread.
—19th century saying

An apple a day, no doctor to pay.
—20th century saying

An apple a day keeps the doctor away.
—20th and 21st century saying

Contents

Chapter 1
Food for Thought on Cancer

Cancer can be as simple as a vitamin deficiency or as complicated as getting exposed to daily chemicals or too much deadly radiation. Which vitamin is it that you are missing? More on that subject later, but I can tell you it's one you won't find on the shelves of your local pharmacy or big box store. If cancer prevention is as simple as adding a vitamin to your diet, then why isn't it available at the stores? Ponder that question as you read on.

It is estimated approximately 40 percent of the individuals living in the United States will develop cancer within the next two decades. This amounts to one hundred and thirty million people. What about all of the advanced X-ray machines, chemotherapy medications, and cancer research dollars collected? One has to ask, why aren't they successful? There's money to be made, so why cure cancer? If you can keep someone alive, but not cured, you can make a mint off of that person. Even if researchers do cure all cancer types, you know the cost will be exorbitant. It's time to take control of your health and minimize your risk of getting cancer.

Dr. Bernadine P. Healy, the first woman to head the National Institutes of Health, which includes the National Cancer Institute, died at the age of 67 of brain cancer. Why does our medical establishment not teach doctors how to cure cancer? Unfortunately, doctors are only taught to focus on the end result—tumors—and not boosting the immune system. The only treatment options allowed by law are chemotherapy, radiation, or surgery—all of which only suppress the immune system and allow the cancer to spread.

Someone I know has had prostate cancer for the last ten years. Doctors gave him a hormone shot on a periodic basis for ten years at $6,000 each. Why would doctors cure you if they can make a profit off of you for ten years? Right? I went into the nearest pharmacy, plucked something off the shelf that I had researched ten minutes on the Internet, and bought it for this man. A month later, he told me his numbers were the lowest they had ever been. It was more effective than all of those shots over the last decade. What is wrong with this picture? So, do you want to put all of your eggs in one basket, or do you want to know what your options are to hedge your bets? If so, you've come to the right location. Someone or something has guided you to be reading this book for a reason.

A cancer diagnosis is shocking. What do you do next? Time is of the essence. You have to get your affairs in order because you don't know the outcome. You trust the medical community and put all of your faith in "the system" for a cure. You feel helpless. You are restricted to the choices of what the medical community is limited to offering by law. Pick your demise.

Radiation therapy does physical damage to the body and destroys your white blood cells, the body's front line defense against cancer. Chemotherapy cannot differentiate between cancerous cells and healthy cells so it destroys your immune system, leaving you open to more health problems, leaving you exhausted. Chemotherapy is only 2.1 percent effective overall in the United States and 2.3 percent effective in Australia, according to researchers at the Department of Radiation Oncology at the Northern Sydney Cancer Centre. The study was based on 154,971 cancer patients treated with conventional cancer treatments.

Why not build up the body's immune system and let it destroy the cancerous cells and leave the healthy cells alone? Well, you can't do it by eating highly processed foods that we have been led to believe are perfectly fine for us and are the normal way to eat.

You must win this cancer battle with every option you can get your hands on. Why wait for a diagnosis? It's much easier to prevent cancer than it is to cure it once you are diagnosed. You can take matters into your own hands and not totally rely on the medical establishment that knows very little about nutrition. As Wendell Berry, an environmental activist stated, "People are fed by the FOOD industry, which pays no attention to HEALTH … and are treated by the HEALTH industry, which pays no attention to FOOD."

The World Health Organization stated that up to 30 percent of all cancers are preventable by avoiding key risk factors such as: tobacco use, being overweight, unhealthy diets, and a lack of physical activity. Cancer has four main contributing factors: environmental toxins (pollution, black mold, asbestos, chemicals, petroleum, fracking chemicals, electric and magnetic fields, radiation, smoking, etc.), stress, hormones, and diet/lifestyle (lack of nutrition in the food due to overprocessing, pesticides, herbicides, hormones like estrogen, growth hormones added to our meat, chemicals, physical inactivity, obesity, excess alcohol use, tanning bed use, etc.).

If we can grow our own food or eat organic foods and they haven't been adulterated with destructive modifications, pesticides, herbicides, and other environmental toxins, then they are probably okay to eat. However, if the foods have been processed and preserved, you might want to think twice about what you are putting in your mouth and the mouths of your children and family.

A man found an old winter coat he had once stashed in his closet about fifteen years earlier. He was checking his pockets and found a hamburger wrapped in wax paper from a popular fast food chain. The burger didn't look a day old except that the lettuce was a little wilted and the bun had cracked just a bit. How many preservatives does it take to keep a burger and bun without mold for fifteen years? Do you really want to eat that, let alone feed that to your children? How are their bodies supposed to grow and keep healthy off food like that? We've been indoctrinated into thinking that highly processed fast food is just the normal modus operandi until some major health scare makes us rethink that strategy.

Wild animals generally don't contract cancer unless they are forced to eat unhealthy foods that man provides in captivity. Many tribal communities around the world rarely get cancer. Why? Their diet consists of caribou or other four-legged animals that eat nitriloside-rich grasses such as Johnson grass, Tunis grass, or Sudan grass. Many grasses contain seventeen thousand milligrams of nitriloside per kilogram of dry weight. Nitriloside is also known as vitamin B17, a natural barrier against cancer growth. Many seeds and berries also contain vitamin B17.

In the computer field, we have a saying "garbage in, garbage out." Whatever crappy data you feed into the computer program will come out as crappy data. The same thing happens when you feed your body highly processed food. All of the nutrition is stripped out of it, leaving your body with nothing to use to support your immune system and eventually something gives out. Imagine taking chemotherapy while eating junk food. It's just like never getting an oil change in your vehicle; eventually the engine seizes up, and the show is over. I want you to think about what goes in your mouth from now on.

Food and drink acidity also can play a huge role in cancer, which we will discuss more in-depth in Chapter 4. Also, a new threat has reached our shores and has landed in the food and on the clothing, jewelry, and products we use on a daily basis. It comes from the radiation expelled from the nuclear power plant disabled by a tsunami in Fukushima, Japan, in 2011. It's time to buy a radiation detector. More information on this threat will be discussed in Chapter 3.

Doctors fear the ability to handle the increase in the number of cancer patients in the future. They expect cuts to government health plans and cuts in payments to doctors. While costs increase and the population ages, the American Society of Clinical Oncology expects cancer to become the No. 1 killer in the United States by the year 2030. That is exactly why you need to read this book and be prepared if you want to have any chance in the fight against cancer for you and your loved ones.

Cancer

In 1879, E.H. Dyer opened the first sugar beet factory in the United States. In the early 1900s, one in twenty people developed cancer. In the 1940s, one in sixteen people developed cancer. In 1957, Richard O. Marshall and Earl R. Kooi invented the production of high fructose corn syrup. In the 1970s, one in ten people were inflicted with cancer. In 1974, the U. S. Food and Drug Administration (FDA) approved the use of aspartame for use in dry foods. It reversed that decision the next year when a psychiatrist claimed it caused brain damage in animals. In 1975, high fructose corn syrup was rapidly incorporated into highly processed foods and soft drinks in the United States.

Today, one in three of us will develop cancer. In 1981, aspartame received approval from the FDA once again. In 1998, the FDA approved sucralose (Splenda®) for use in the United States. The number of people with a cancer history in the United States has dramatically increased from three million in the early 1970s to almost fourteen million today in 2016. A Midwest oncologist (a cancer doctor) stated that cancer feeds off of sugar. Sixty-eight percent of today's cancer patients were given their diagnoses since 2010. More than 50 percent of the cancer survivors are over the age of 64. Increased survival rates are due to early screening, improved treatment options, better cancer drugs, prevention methodologies, and targeted therapies. More people are developing cancer, but the death rates are falling. Cancer is big business.

Cells are the basic building block of every tissue in the body. We have different types of cells that have specific functions, such as blood, brain, and skin cells. When these cells change, mutate, or divide abnormally and deviate from their specific function, that is when cancer begins. This change makes the cells grow out of control, forming a tumor.

What causes cancer? Genetics, lack of nutrition in our diet, too much sun exposure, too much sugar, sexual transmission, obesity, age, and exposure to environmental toxins, too many hormones (from food or shots), radiation, and tobacco use can all be causes of cancer.

Drs. Rainer Klement and Ulrike Kammerer published literature connecting dietary carbohydrates to cancer cells in the October 2011 journal *Nutrition and Metabolism*. They concluded that increasing glucose allows cancer to proliferate and spread. Eating white sugar, refined flour, and processed foods creates a magnesium mineral deficiency in the body, and deficiencies in magnesium allow cancer to flourish. Cut off the supply of sugar, and cancer is suppressed.

Food for Thought

How much sugar are you ingesting each day? The World Health Organization recommends no more than twenty-five grams, or six teaspoons per day. Your body has to work hard to process sugar and receives no nutrition in return. Take yogurt, for example. Let's say that one container contains twenty-six grams of sugar. Approximately four grams of sugar are in one regular sugar cube. So, in twenty-six grams of yogurt, you have six-and-one-half sugar cubes. Now, let's say you have one container of yogurt a day. That amounts to 2,372.5 sugar cubes a year. How many other food products are you ingesting that contain sugar each day? What about cereal? Many brands contain approximately eighteen grams of sugar per two-thirds cup serving. Let's say you have two servings for breakfast. The total amounts to nine sugar cubes, or thirty-six grams. Multiply that for our annual consumption, and it totals 3,285 sugar cubes. Let's add that to the annual yogurt count, and you have 5,657.5 sugar cubes. Add a daily twenty-ounce bottle of soda (sixty-five grams / sixteen-and-a-quarter cubes), and you have 5,931.25 sugar cubes, plus the yogurt and cereal counts, equals 11,588.75 sugar cubes—or 53 pounds of sugar each year! Do you see the picture? And we wonder why diabetes, heart disease, and cancer are on the rise? An excellent article "Cancer's Sweet Tooth" can be found at mercola.com.

The average consumption of sugar in the United States in 1887 was five pounds per person per year. Now, the average consumption is five pounds in two weeks. Currently, almost thirteen million people globally are diagnosed with cancer each year and almost sixty percent die from cancer. Cancer is the second leading cause of death in the United States. The No. 1 cause is heart disease, according to the American Cancer Society. Heart disease is linked to an increase in fructose consumption.

Why wait for a cancer diagnosis? There are many steps that you can undertake now to lower your risk of getting cancer. Many people say, "I don't have the time to cook" or "I don't have the money to eat organic." Do you have time to sit in the hospital for weeks or months on end dealing with an endless parade of surgeons, radiologists, and/or oncologists? One chemotherapy treatment can take up to three hours. Do you have $50,000 or more to spend on cancer treatments and/or other hospital expenses? One chemotherapy drug on an outpatient basis can cost $26,000. Many report that each round of chemotherapy costs $10,000, with six rounds required. Depending on how many times you go through it, you could be in the $100,000 range. Prostate cancer may require a shot of medicine that costs $6,000 for each shot. Some hospitals have a facility fee of approximately $2,000 just for setting foot in their facility. It doesn't include medications or seeing a doctor or nurse.

Don't forget the maintenance that comes after you have cancer. The financial burden, on average, for cancer survivors is $8,000 a year for men and $8,400 a year for women. Plus, add in $4,000 for productivity loss. That will buy a lot of organic food. Many lose thousands of dollars in productivity from lost work hours, and many even quit their jobs. One-third of cancer survivors have had to limit their daily activities. Currently, there are more than thirteen million cancer survivors in the United States. That number is expected to rise to eighteen million in the near future. The American Cancer Society reports 49,000 Americans will be diagnosed with pancreatic cancer in a year and more than 40,000 will die of it.

The Swedish Environmental Research Institute (IVL) studied whether changing to organic foods would lower the levels of pesticides found in people's bodies. The study was performed on a family of five. Researchers had family members eat their regular diets for a week while testing their urine. The next two weeks, the family ate organic foods only, followed by daily testing of their urine. The average pesticide levels were reduced by a factor of 9.5. Here is a list of the pesticides, herbicides, fungicides, and insecticides that were found in their bodies:

MCPA (herbicide)
Ethylenebisdithiocarbamates (fungicide)
Atrazine (herbicide)
Chlorpyrifos (insecticide)
Thiabendazole, iprodione, diuron, vinclozolin (fungicides)
Boscalid (fungacide)
2,4-dichlorophenoxyacetic acid (herbicides)
Pyrethroids, such as cypermethrin and esfenvalerate (insecticides)
Propamocarb (fungicide)
Chlormequat chloride (CCC) and mepequat (growth inhibitors)

The mother of the family stated, "Overall, you think about the kids. There were a whole number of chemicals removed from my kids' bodies. And I don't want them back."

MCPA symptoms in humans range from slurred speech, twitching, jerking and spasms, drooling, low blood pressure, and unconsciousness.

Ethylenebisdithiocarbamates cause irritation of the skin, respiratory tract, and eyes. Prolonged exposure can lead to chronic skin diseases. This chemical has a wide range of uses, including treatment of blights on tomatoes and potatoes, vegetables, fruit, commercial sod, and other crops.

Atrazine is known as a weed killer. It is used on sugarcane, corn, pineapples, sorghum, macadamia nuts, and evergreen farm trees. Exposure to fetuses can cause low fetal weight and heart, urinary, and limb defects. In animals, it causes liver, kidney, and heart damage. (See page 77 for an alternative weed killer recipe.)

Chlorpyrifos is a highly toxic pesticide once used in the United States nerve toxin, chlorpyrifos has been associated with birth defects, neurological injuries, and ailments. It is used on fruits and vegetables.

Thiabendazole, iprodione, diuron, vinclozolin fungicides cause cancer, developmental problems, reproductive problems, endocrine disruption, immunotoxicity, and neurotoxicity. They also cause toxicity to skin, sense organs, cardiovascular systems, blood, stomach, intestines, liver, kidney, and respiratory systems. They are likely to cause cancer.

Boscalid targets the toxicity in the liver. It has induced thyroid tumors in rats. It is used as a fungicide for canola, legumes, fruit, and vegetable crops.

Cypermethrin mainly affects the nervous and muscular systems. Symptoms include uncoordinated movements, exaggerated reaction to stimuli, trembling or shaking movements, skin sensations of tingling, tickling, or prickling, lethargy, fatigue, vomit, diarrhea, and urinary incontinence. Cypermethrin is used in crop pesticides and in public or domestic hygiene as a biocide.

Propamocarbs have been tested on laboratory animals, and studies show decreased body weight gain and decreased motor activity. Females experienced a weight gain. Males had a decreased sperm count, motility, and abnormal sperm morphology. Salivation, reddish material around the mouth, and urine staining are common. Offspring effects include death, decreased viability, smaller litter sizes, smaller sizes, and weight issues.

Chlormequat chloride is moderately toxic. In animal laboratory studies, skin, eye, oral tests were administered. Moderate oral and dermal toxicity was found. Also in animal studies, diarrhea, vomiting, salvation, reduced body weight, down-growth of the ovaries, and endometrial hyperplasia in mice were found. It was not found to be carcinogenic in rats and mice. It is used in wheat, rye, oats, and triticale. Also it is used on cotton and flowering azaleas, fuchsias, begonias, poinsettias, pelargoniums, and other ornamental plants.

Still think you can't afford organic food? It has been scientifically proven that organic food has more nutrition than genetically modified food. You can shop for organics that are on sale and stock up. It doesn't have to break your budget. You can work your recipes around what is on sale at the time. Plant organic tomato or potato plants in buckets, large pots, or barrels with drainage holes. Create a raised garden bed or just till up a spot in your back yard. Plant some garlic and onions in a large pot or spread them in with other plants. They can even go in between plants in the same row. They also help to keep bugs and underground critters away.

Did you know that when you eat fresh garlic and raw onions, mosquitoes stay away for four to five hours, and no chemicals have to be absorbed into your skin? Garlic and onions are great cancer, virus, and bacteria fighters. Keep this in mind with mosquito infestations in the news.

Pet Cancer

Dog cancer can cost anywhere from $200 to $15,000 if it requires chemotherapy, radiation, and surgery. Bone marrow transplants can be very expensive for lymphoma cancer.

Cat cancer can range from $200 to around $5,000 or more. Many may require a treatment plan that will last up to six months.

You may want to discuss your pet's diet, nutrition, and exercise plans with your veterinarian. See the following chapter for more information on pet cancer.

Chapter 2
Cancer Symptoms in People and Pets

Many of the most common cancer symptoms in men are an abnormal lump under the skin, a change in testicles, changes in bowel and bladder habits, changes in your skin such as blisters, bleeding, scaling, moles, sores, or mutating freckles, indigestion or trouble swallowing, persistent cough, mouth changes such as white patches, sores, bleeding, numbness or tenderness, unexplained weight loss, fatigue, back pain, headache, abdominal pain or stomach pains.

Women should watch for breast changes, bloating, weight loss or bleeding, between-period bleeding, skin changes such as a mutating mole, blood in your stool, changes in your lymph nodes, trouble swallowing, heartburn, mouth changes such as white or bright red patches, a fever that doesn't go away, fatigue, cough, ongoing pain, belly pain, or depression.

In general, signs of cancer are unexplained weight loss, fever, extreme fatigue, pain, skin changes, change in bowel habits, changes in bladder functions, sores that won't heal, white oral patches, unusual bleeding, lumps, indigestion or trouble swallowing, wart or mole changes, nagging cough or hoarseness.

Symptoms for childhood acute lymphoblastic leukemia are bone and joint pain, fatigue, weakness, bleeding, fever, and weight loss. Brain tumors can cause headaches, dizziness, frequent vomiting, balance problems, and vision, hearing, or speech problems.

Neuroblastoma results from cells that haven't matured in infants and young children, and the symptoms can be impaired walking, changes in eyes such as bulging, dark circles, and droopy eyelids, pain in various locations in the body, diarrhea, and high blood pressure. Wilms tumors usually start in one kidney and are found in young children under age six. They can cause swelling or a lump in the belly, fever, pain, nausea, and a poor appetite.

Childhood lymphoma starts in the immune system. The cancers affect lymph nodes and other lymph tissues such as the tonsils or thymus. The bone marrow also can be affected. Lymphoma symptoms consist of swollen lymph nodes in the neck, armpit, or groin, weight loss, fever, sweats, and weakness.

If these symptoms are present, it doesn't necessarily mean that you have cancer. You should consult your doctor or pediatrician if the symptoms are persistent or if you have any questions.

Dog Cancer

Symptoms of cancer for dogs can be lumps, swelling, persistent sores, abnormal discharge anywhere from the body, bad breath, sleepiness, rapid weight loss, sudden lameness, dark tarry stools, loss of appetite, difficulty breathing, urinating, or defecating.

Indoor second-hand and outdoor smoke can contribute to the chances of your pet getting cancer.

Make sure your dog has frequent access to fresh pesticide-free grass. Grass contains nitriloside, which is a cancer killer. (More on this later.)

Cat Cancer

Cancer symptoms for cats can range from a lump that changes size or shape to a sore that does not heal. A change in bowel or bladder habits, difficulty eating, swallowing, urinating, or defecating also can be signs. Many will exhibit unexplained bleeding or a discharge from the body as well as a loss of appetite and chronic weight loss.

Environmental factors also can be a factor in your pet's health. Our dog drank water from a field that had been sprayed and suffered from it. Second-hand smoke and licking the body that has been in contact with an environmental toxin also can be contributing causes. Outdoor smoke also can contribute to the chances of your pet getting cancer.

If your dog or cat exhibits any of these symptoms, you should contact your veterinarian immediately. You also may want to consider consulting a veterinary cancer specialist.

Make sure your cat also has access to fresh, pesticide-free grass. Grass contains nitriloside, which is a cancer killer. (More on this later.)

Pet Toxins

Here are just a few of the pet toxins you should be aware of and keep away from your pet: chocolate, apple seeds, insect bait stations, rodenticides (mouse and rat poisons), fertilizers, field sprays for weeds, xylitol (found in sugar-free gums and candies), ibuprofen (Advil™ or Motrin™ or their generic form), acetaminophen (Tylenol™ or generic form), silica gel packs, amphetamines such as ADD or ADHD drugs, and household cleaners.

A few pet-friendly recipes have been included in the Miscellaneous recipe section in Chapter 9.

Chapter 3
Nuclear Radiation

Since the earthquake in Japan of March 2011, and the collapse of the Fukushima nuclear power plant, nuclear radiation has reportedly reached the shores of California, and it is starting to infiltrate our food supply, as well as imported products from overseas. For example, coral calcium is harvested in the Pacific Ocean, and it is polluted with radiation. Manufacturers crush the coral and use it in all kinds of coral calcium products that have originated off the shores of Japan, such as vitamins, calcium children's chewable vitamins, other supplements, and water filters that add alkalinity to your water. Calcium-based powder also is used on plastic food storage bags and plastic food containers to keep them from sticking together. My family has switched to reusable bpa-free containers. Fish also have been found to have higher radioactive levels near the western shores of the United States.

When I researched coral calcium manufacturers one major manufacturer was listed out of Okinawa, Japan. There are other manufacturers located in other oceans besides the Pacific Ocean.

We have found that nuts from Asia are now polluted with radiation. We bought an organic container of mixed nuts and berries. When the list of origin of the nuts listed China, we tested the container, and it showed up with radiation. Sea salt also may be radioactive if manufactured near the Pacific Ocean. However, there are many sea salt manufacturers, not all of them are located on the West Coast. Online, we have read that nuts, prunes, and sardines now contain low trace amounts of radiation. Keep in mind that the instructions that came with our particular radiation detector stated that there are, "no safe levels of nuclear radiation."

Make sure you wash anything you bring home from China or Japan before eating it, wearing it, or using it. You have to look out for yourself.

So, the government has raised the amount of radiation that is allowable in our food. How much is too much? Experts say low amounts are harmless, but some studies say about 5 percent of the people exposed to low doses of radiation will end up dying from cancer. One doctor claims that one hundred X-rays is a lifetime limit with the non-digital X-rays. Medical facilities purchase expensive equipment to take X-rays and they want to use it and get their money's worth. One machine may cost upwards of three million dollars. A big hospital or clinic may have several units.

Newer digital X-ray machines offer a lower dose of radiation, but technicians can potentially produce more images than needed or produce higher quality images than required, which creates an increase in the dosage.

I told my dentist I didn't want any X-rays for a while. They looked at me like I was an alien. I waited three years and then they took about eight X-rays. Wouldn't three suffice (front, left side, and right side)? What is the worst thing that happens if I don't get my teeth X-rayed? I lose a tooth. What is the worst thing that happens if I get eight X-rays every other year, which is what they want to do? I could incur potential damage to bone, blood, or the brain. By the time I'm 75, I would have been X-rayed 300 times. Add in mammograms (which have an 11 percent false-positive rate) for twenty-five years, and now I'm up to 500 X-rays, assuming I don't have any CAT scans. Break an arm or leg bone? Add another 50 to 70 X-rays. Need braces on your teeth? Add even more, including a whole head X-ray. And is that too much radiation? We are way over the 100 lifetime limit recommended by one doctor. Every X-ray permanently damages living tissue, which accumulates in the body. Supposedly, new digital X-rays are one-tenth the dose of the old film X-rays.

One of the discoverers of radium, Marie Curie, died of radiation-induced leukemia in 1934. What part of that sounded like a good idea to mass-produce machines that irradiate our bodies when the inventor died from it? Excuse me?! And what part of creating nuclear power plants in earthquake-prone zones sounded like a good idea, especially when we have no idea on how to deal with the irradiated waste?

"Theoretically, even the smallest amount of radiation could contribute to cancer induction," says George Casarett, a member of the Nuclear Regulatory Commission. Small amounts taken in year after year become dangerous and may take decades to show up as radiation-induced tumors.

The three types of nuclear radiation we are researching here are alpha, beta, and gamma. Alpha is the lightest version of radiation, where a piece of paper can stop the rays. Beta can be stopped with a thin metal sheet or aluminum. Thick lead or steel plates can stop gamma or X-rays. However, neutron radiation is the most deadliest. It can go through lead and can only be stopped by large amounts of water or concrete.

Alpha particles can travel several millimeters in the air but their distance decreases with the density of matter. These particles cannot penetrate human skin, but if inhaled, alpha particles can damage lung tissue. Many radiation detectors do not detect this type of radiation, which is now reportedly being brought into our country on products from countries where radiation accidents have occurred.

Beta particles are much lighter and can travel farther. One particle, on average, travels one meter by air and one millimeter in body tissue.

Gamma rays may be emitted in bundles called photons if the decay is in an excited state. Gamma particles are electromagnetic radiation and can penetrate deeper than alpha or beta particles. Many gamma rays can pass through a person's body without affecting the tissue at all, and others can ionize atoms in your tissue. It's like standing next to an active volcano and having a ball of lava pass through your body, cauterizing as it goes, only on a much smaller, still harmful, level.

Radiation is measured in different units, depending on the country you are in and their standards. Over the past century, the Curie (Ci), Rad, and Rem were developed. With the metric system, the Becquerel (Bq), Sievert, and Gray—otherwise known as the System Internationale (SI)—was developed by scientists. For the dose of radiation given off by material that is radioactive, the term curie is used and the SI unit Becquerel. Becquerel is equivalent to a radioactive decay rate of one disintegration per second. For the amount of radiation absorbed by a person, the term rad and the SI unit Gray is used. For the potential risk of exposure of radiation, the unit rem and the SI unit Sievert is used.

1 microSiever (µSv) = 0.1 mrem
1 milliSievert (mSv) = 100 mrem
1 centiSievert (cSv) = 1 rem (1000 millirem)
1 Sievert (Sv) = 100 rem
1 Gray (Gy) = 100 Rads = 1 Sievert (Sv) = 100 Rem

Conversion factors between the two units are as follows:
1 Ci = 3.7×1010 Bq (37 billion Becquerels)
1 Ci = 37 GBq (37 GigaBecquerels)
1 µCi = 37,000 Bq
1 Bq = 2.70×10-11 Ci (less than one ten billionth of a Curie)
1 Bq = 2.70×10-5 µCi
1 GBq = 0.0270 Ci

According to the U.S. Nuclear Regulatory Commission (www.nrc.gov), if an individual were in an area where radiation was continuously present, the dose should not exceed 0.002 rem or 0.02 mSv in an hour and 0.05 rem or 0.5 mSv in a year.

If radionuclide concentrations were inhaled or ingested continuously over the course of a year, it would produce a dose of 0.05 rem (50 millrem or 0.5 millisieverts). (A radionuclide is an atom or nucleus that is radioactive.) The probability of radiation-induced cancer increases by 5 to 6 percent for every 1,000 mSv of dose.

Exposure examples:
Exposure to cosmic rays during a roundtrip airplane flight from New York to Los Angeles—3 mrem 0.03 mSv
One dental X-ray—4 to 15 mrem or 0.04 to 0.15 mSv
One bitewing X-ray—0.038 mSv
Full mouth X-ray—0.15 mSv
Panoramic X-ray—0.005 to 0.01 mSv
One chest X-ray—8 to 10 mrem or 0.08 to 0.1 mSv
One chest CT scan—1 to 16 mSv

One mammogram—40 to 70 mrem or 0.04 to 0.7 mSv
Pelvis/hip/abdomen X-ray—60 to 70 mrem or 0.6 to 0.7 mSv
Knee/other extremities X-ray—0.001 to 0.005 mSv
Thoracic Spine/lumbar spine X-ray—1.0 to 1.5 mSv
Skull X-ray—0.1 mSv
Head/neck CT scan—2 to 3 mSv
One year of exposure to natural radiation (from soil, cosmic rays, etc.)—
   300 mrem or 3 mSv
Brick, concrete—0.1 to 0.2 mSv/year
Natural stone, technically produced gypsum—0.2 to 0.4 mSv/year
Slag brick, granite (some countertops, flooring)—0.4 to 2 mSv/year

Vintage Orange to Red Dishware and Radon Gas

Scientific research shows bright orange to red Fiesta dishware can give off radon gas and radiation. When people think about radon testing in homes, they usually think about it coming from the ground, but Fiesta ceramics made before 1972 should always be considered suspect. The bright orange/red dishware became radioactive from the uranium-based paints used in the manufacturing process.

Radon is a radioactive gas caused from normal decay of uranium, thorium, and radium in rocks and soil. It can seep into a house through cracks in the foundation or ground water. Radon can cause lung cancer.

Vintage Vaseline Glass

Uranium oxide was added to green glassware, making it radioactive with a low dosage. One way to tell if a piece is radioactive is to put the glassware under a black light. If radioactive, it will fluoresce (glow).

Dinosaur Bones

Have you ever been to a museum where there are dinosaur bones on display? Ever notice they are painted a dark color? The paint is lead-based to prevent the radiation from leaking. Why are dinosaur bones radioactive? Some scientists cite elemental uranium deposits in the western United States as the culprit. However, not all bones are from the West.

Some scientists at NASA and the University of Kansas suspect that gamma-ray bursts from nearby stars in our galaxy may have caused the mass extinctions of dinosaurs by damaging Earth's ozone layer. All it takes is just one ten-second burst to cause years of devastating damage.

So, if you want to go on a scavenger hunt for dinosaur bones, just take your Geiger counter with you and wear protective masks and clothing.

A recommended LiveStrong video on youtube.com is, "Cancer is Not a Cell It's a Fungus (Candida), Preventative care is Deathcare in Sheep's Clothing."

Chapter 4
Food pH Charts

"Let food be thy medicine and medicine be thy food" —Hippocrates

The foods listed in this chapter reflect their acidic or alkalizing effects on the body when ingested. For example, when citrus fruits are eaten, they become alkalizing inside the body and thus very beneficial. A healthy balance is 20 percent acidic and 80 percent alkaline foods.

Your body is designed to be healthy in an alkaline state of a pH level of 7.4 or higher. At this level, cancer cells become dormant and at a pH of 8.5 and up, the cancer cells will die and healthy cells live. Correct oxygen levels in the body will also help to neutralize acidity. When your body is too acidic (a low pH number), it prevents the oxygen from reaching the body tissues. When cells are lacking oxygen, the acidity levels rise (6.0 pH or lower) and can make dormant cancer cells become active. See more information at the Complete Health and Happiness website, "The Root Cause of Cancer and Why Has it Been Kept a Secret!"

Keep in mind that thirty-two cups of alkaline water are needed to neutralize one cup of pop or soda. Imagine what that does to your body when you drink a super-sized sugary drink. When your body becomes too acidic, it cannot fight off diseases, colds, flus, cancer, and a whole host of other illnesses. Sugar offers nothing to the body of nutritional value and therefore your body has to expend energy to deal with processing an overload of sugar. This stresses the body until your health suffers.

The food pH chart starts at 2.5 pH (very acidic) and ends with a 10 pH (very alkaline). Remember, raw fruits and vegetables are the best. By cooking the food, it becomes more acidic. In general, it takes twenty or more parts of alkalinity to neutralize one part acidity in the body.

Considerable variations can exist in pH levels depending on the variety of produce, growing conditions, and processing methods.

Acidic Foods and Beverages (Recommended 20% of your diet)

Miscellaneous:
Optimum pH for human blood is 7.365

2.5 pH
Beverages:
Colas

2.86 pH
Lemon Brisk in a can

2.96 pH
Lemon Nestea

3.0 pH
Meats:
Bacon
Pork
Sausages

Dairy:
Processed cheeses

Sweets:
Pudding

Miscellaneous:
Aspartame
Equal
French fries
Fried foods
NutraSweet®
Overwork
Regular vinegar
Sleep deprivation
Stress
Sweet 'N Low®
Tobacco Smoke
Worry
Yeast

3.2 pH
Light-colored soda/pop

3.5 pH
Meats:
Canned tuna
Lobster

Dairy:
Ice cream

Nuts:
Most roasted nuts
Hazelnuts

Beverages:
Carbonated soft drinks (except colas)
Sugarized grapefruit juice
Sugarized orange juice

Fats and Oils:
Cottonseed oil
Palm oil

4.0 pH
Vegetables:
Most legumes
Snow peas
Tomato sauce

Meats:
Veal

Dairy:
Buttermilk
Cream cheese

Grains:
Granola
White bread
Flour tortillas

Sweets:
Artificial sweeteners

Miscellaneous:
Peanuts
White vinegar

4.5 pH
Vegetables:
Sorrel

Meats:
Beef
Pork
Mussels
Squid
Other mollusks

Dairy:
Goat cheese

Pasta:
White pasta

Beverages:
Most beers
Black teas
Hard liquor
Most coffee
Sugary fruit juices

Sweets:
Jams and jellies
Pastries made from white flour
    and sugar
White sugar

Miscellaneous:
Most microwave foods
Unsweetened cocoa

5.0 pH
Vegetables:
Most frozen vegetables
Most canned vegetables
Cooked Swiss chard
Navy beans

Meats:
Most wild game

Dairy:
Cottage cheese

Grains:
Barley
Oat bran
Rice cakes

Beverages:
Most wine

Sweets:
Stevia

Miscellaneous:
Balsamic vinegar
Cigarettes
Iodized table salt

5.5 pH
Fruits:
Pomegranate

Vegetables:
Garbanzo beans
Lima beans

Meats:
Chicken
Turkey
Duck
Goose
Lamb
Goat
Venison
Elk

Grains:
Processed cereals
Rice white semolina
Wheat bran
White flour
Wheat flour

Nuts:
Brazil nuts
Walnuts
Pecans

Fats and Oils:
Sesame oil
Safflower oil
Almond oil

Beverages:
Reverse osmosis filtered water
Bottled water
Sports drinks

Sweets:
Brown sugar
Chocolate
Custard with white sugar
Sweetened yogurt
Tapioca

Miscellaneous:
Ketchup
Jar mayonnaise
Mustard
Vanilla
Most pharmaceutical drugs

6.0 pH
Fruits:
Dates
Figs
Dried fruits
Cooked cranberries
Prunes

Vegetables:
Red beetroots
Black-eyed peas
Peeled potatoes
Most pickles
Cooked zucchini

Meats:
Salmon
Tuna
Other fish
Oysters
Shellfish

Dairy:
Plain yogurt

Grains:
Corn bread
Tortillas
Cream of wheat
Most whole grain breads
Popcorn with salt and butter
Rye germ
Wheat germ
Wheat germ

Nuts:
Pistachios
Pine nuts

Beverages:
Kona coffee
Soy milk
Rice milk
Almond milk

Fats and Oils:
Salted butter
Pumpkin oil
Grape seed oil

Sweets:
Processed maple syrup
Sulphured molasses

Miscellaneous:
Gelatin
Hummus

6.5 pH
Fruits:
Green bananas
Plums

Vegetables:
Cooked green peas
Horseradish
Kidney and pinto beans
Pickled olives
Cooked spinach

Meats:
Cooked whole eggs and egg whites
Liver
Other organ meats

Dairy:
Processed cow and goat milk
Processed dairy products
Most cheeses

Grains:
Oats
Buckwheat
Corn and rice breads
Cornmeal
Buttered popcorn with no salt
Sprout breads
Sunflower seeds
Wheat crackers
Rye crackers
Rice crackers
Whole grain

Miscellaneous:
Cashew milk (A few websites say
     slightly acidic but most say alkaline)
Rice vinegar
Soy cheese
Soy sauce

Sweets:
Carob
Fructose
Pastries with honey
Pastries with whole grain

Neutral Foods and Beverages
7.0 pH
Meats:
Egg yolks cooked soft

Dairy:
Unsalted butter and margarine
Raw cow milk
Raw goat milk
Raw cow whey
Raw goat whey
Raw cream

Grains:
Brown and basmati rice

Beverages:
Municipal tap water

Fats and Oils:
Canola oil
Corn oil
Sunflower oil

Sweets:
Barley malt syrup
Raw honey

Alkaline Foods and Beverages (Improves body acidity) (Recommended 80% of your diet)

7.5 pH

Fruits:
Blueberries
Fresh coconut
Raw cranberries
Fresh guava and sapote
Strawberries

Vegetables:
Bamboo shoots
Beets without greens
Chives
Cooked Brussels sprouts
Cooked broccoli
Cooked squash
Cooked eggplant
Fresh corn
Cooked kale
Cooked soybeans
Okra
Potatoes with skins
Radishes
Tofu

Grains:
Flax seeds
Millet
Spelt
Quinoa

Nuts:
Chestnuts

Beverages:
Unprocessed apple cider
Grain coffee substitutes

Fats and Oils:
Flax oil
Avocado oil
Primrose oil

Sweets:
Raw maple syrup

Miscellaneous:
Homemade mayonnaise
Sea salt
Tamari sauce

8.0 pH

Fruits:
Apples
Canteloupe
Cherries
Currants
Gooseberries
Ripe bananas
Fresh oranges
Fresh peaches
Tomatoes

Vegetables:
Arrowroot
Avocados
Bell pepper
Cauliflower
Fresh mushrooms
Fresh pumpkin
Fresh ripe olives
Fresh tomato
Jicama
Kohlrabi
Parsnip
Raw green cabbage
Rhubarb
Soybeans
Turnips
Turnip greens

Grains:
Sesame seeds
Wild rice

Nuts:
Organic almonds
Almond butter

Beverages:
Natural unsweetened fruit juices
Sake

Fats and Oils:
Fish oil

Sweets:
Unsulphured molasses

Miscellaneous:
Fresh herbs
Fresh spices
Miso soup
Vegetable sea salt
Apple cider vinegar
Conch (7.5 to 8.0)

8.5 pH (a pH of 8.5 to 10 is reportedly able to kill cancer cells)
Fruits:
Blackberries
Cantaloupe
Honeydew melons
Most melons
Fresh apricots
Fresh dates
Fresh figs
Grapefruit
Grapes
Kiwi
Nectarine
Fresh pears
Papaya
Passion fruit
Raisins

Vegetables:
Alfalfa
Other sprouted grains
Carrots
Fresh garlic
Fresh ginger
Fresh ginseng
Green beans
Kudzu root
Most lettuces
Leaks
Rutabagas
Taro root
Fresh sweet peas

Beverages:
Ginger tea
Mu tea

Miscellaneous:
Cayenne
Cinnamon

9.0 pH (a pH of 8.5 to 10 is reportedly able to kill cancer cells)
Fruits:
Loganberries
Persimmons
Fresh mangoes
Papayas
Pineapple
Fresh raspberries
Tangerines
Umeboshi plums

Vegetables:
Alfalfa sprouts
Artichokes
Beets with greens
Raw celery
Raw cucumber
Endive

Raw eggplant
Sweet potatoes
Yams
Dried soy beans
Unroasted dried pumpkin seeds
Sea vegetables
Watercress
Raw zucchini

Beverages:
Green tea
Herbal tea

Miscellaneous:
Borage oil
Cilantro
Parsley
Stevia plant
Kelp
Karengo
Olive oil
Other seaweed

**9.5 pH (a pH of 8.5 to 10 is
reportedly able to kill cancer cells)
Fruits:**
Watermelon

Vegetables:
Raw broccoli
Straw wheat, lemon, other green
    grasses
Potato skins only
Raw kale
Raw mustard greens

Beverages:
Fresh raw vegetable juices
Blended green grasses drinks
Alkaline water

**10.0 pH (a pH of 8.5 to 10 is
reportedly able to kill cancer cells)
Fruits:**
Fresh lemons
Fresh limes
Vegetables:
Asparagus
Collards
Cucumbers
Onions
Raw red cabbage
Raw Brussels sprouts
Raw Swiss chard
Kimchi
Other fermented vegetables
Raw spinach

Miscellaneous:
Baking soda (I recommend using organic baking soda or one that does not have aluminum in it. This can be ordered online if it is not available in your area. One source is www.frontiercoop.com).

Eat colorful vegetables and fruits for your health.

White vegetables and fruits
    strengthen your immune system.
Yellow vegetables and fruits fortify
    your skin's elasticity.
Sugar thins the skin, especially in
    your later years.
Orange vegetables and fruits prevent
    inflammation.
Red vegetables and fruits improve
    your heart and blood health.
Purple vegetables and fruits protect
    your nervous system.
Green vegetables and fruits detoxify
    your body.

Chapter 5
Cold Prevention

One of the most important factors in staying well is to get plenty of sleep. Make an effort to get at least seven to eight hours daily. I see so many people rushing down the interstate in the morning because they didn't get up in time because they didn't go to bed on time. I saw a woman putting mascara on in her rear view mirror driving down the interstate at seventy-plus miles per hour. Get some sleep so you can get up ten minutes earlier and drive normal speeds. If you are chronically getting colds, you are probably lacking sleep and are not eating enough alkaline foods. Check out the pH foods list provided in this book and eat extra foods from the pH of 8-plus, 9-plus, and 10 ranges. I once had a grade school teacher ask why my son never got sick. We minimize sugar intake, we don't drink soda or pop, we eat fresh vegetables and fruits regularly, and we eat protein (fresh fish, fresh chicken, occasional beef, and pork, organic or free range) when at all possible. Your body needs fresh foods (not highly processed) to fight off viruses and infections. Most children eat what is called "beige" foods—crackers, breads, chips, pudding, cheap pasta, cheap pizza, etc.—where everything has no color and it's all highly processed.

Wash your hands frequently during cold and flu season. Try not to touch your head with unwashed hands, especially your eyes, ears, nose, or mouth. Stay home or work from home if you can during the height of cold and flu season. Stock up on two weeks worth of grocery items so you can stay out of the grocery store, minimizing your exposure to illnesses. Use winter gloves when in the grocery store in the winter. This prevents you from touching surfaces that have been contaminated by others with a cold or flu.

If you start to feel just a tinge of achiness in the back of your throat, now is the time to take action. Listen to what your body is telling you. Nip it in the bud. Don't wait until you are sneezing and coughing all over everyone. It's too late then! The cold will have to take its course of two weeks. Take two zinc pills with food at the first sign of a sore throat or achy head feeling. You should take two pills of zinc a day for no more than three days because zinc is a heavy metal and can build up in your body with health consequences. If you can, take a one-hour nap. This is better than anything on the list. Your body's pH becomes acidic with a lack of sleep. By taking a nap, your body becomes more alkaline and can heal itself.

Incorporate one tablespoon of coconut oil in your breakfast (oatmeal, non-sugar smoothie, scrambled eggs, etc.). This is helpful on a regular basis.

Another remedy is to take half a dropper full of elderberry juice extract with a half cup of water. Elderberry anything (pills, juice, or extract) works very well. Take it at the first sign of a cold.

To fight off a sore throat, pour a can of diet ginger ale in a cup, add six dashes of ground ginger. Drink. Within an hour, you will notice the difference. I only recommend diet ginger ale because viruses feed off of sugar. Normally, I don't consume artificial sweeteners. You also can add five to six dashes of ginger in green tea with honey to taste. Green tea leaves contain antioxidants that help boost your immune system. A study by *The Journal of the American College of Nutrition* found people experienced 36 percent fewer sick days when consuming green tea. Steep green tea in six ounces of boiled water for three minutes to maximize the benefits.

I like to take an Advil® Cold & Sinus pill that can be found over-the counter at your local pharmacy. It seems to help in combination with the other non-pill alternatives I will list below.

The Amish swallow two cloves of garlic, one at a time, with food. Garlic acts like a natural antibiotic and antiviral remedy. See Chapter 7.

Buy a NeilMed® Sinus Rinse kit. These kits work great if you feel a sinus headache coming or if you have been working in an area where there is a lot of dust or airborne particulates. I highly suggest buying a gallon of distilled water to use with this kit. Don't use tap water.

Take a one-hour medium-hot bath (don't over do it here, and if you are pregnant or suspect you are, skip this option.) Many people like to add one cup of Epsom salt to their bath.

Honey and Cinnamon to Tackle Colds

1 tablespoon raw honey (organic raw honey, if available)
1/4 teaspoon cinnamon (Use Ceylon cinnamon, if available)

Mix thoroughly. Eat plain or on toast, oatmeal, or cereal. Take once a day for three days. You should see results within a day or two.

Honey and cinnamon are antiviral, antibacterial, and antifungal. This combination also may alleviate bladder and kidney infections, reduce sugar levels, reduce your blood pressure, and help with arthritis pain.

See also the garlic-honey recipe in Chapter 7.

"People are fed by the FOOD industry, which pays no attention to HEALTH … and are treated by the HEALTH industry, which pays no attention to FOOD."

—Wendell Berry
Environmental activist

Sore Throat Remedy

Cup of hot, drinkable water
2 tablespoons honey
2 tablespoons vinegar
2 tablespoons lemon juice
2 dashes cinnamon
6 dashes ground ginger

Mix well and enjoy! You will feel better in short order.

Orange and Coconut Smoothie

1 cup orange juice
1-1/2 cups coconut milk
6 clementine oranges
2 teaspoons raw or dried ginger
2 lemons, juiced
4 tablespoons melted coconut oil
1 cup spinach, tightly packed
1 cup oats (optional)
2 tablespoons chia seeds (optional)
4 tablespoons raw manuka honey (optional)
20 drops of Echinacea (optional)

Blend the first six ingredients until smooth. Add the spinach and blend again. Add optional ingredients one at a time until smooth. Add water to thin out if needed. Makes two servings. Serve daily for best results.

Foods Rich in Vitamin C

Organic strawberries, oranges, sweet red peppers, broccoli, lemons, lime, and grapefruit all help boost your immune system. These foods are all great for your health.

Foods Rich in Iron

Lean, grass-raised red meats and poultry and beans provide iron-rich foods that help fight off infections.

Hydrogen Peroxide and Epsom Salt Detoxification Bath

3 to 4 (16-ounce) bottles of 3% hydrogen peroxide
2 cups Epsom salt

Mix together in a hot water bath. Soak for thirty minutes. Repeat one to three times a week (no vitamins should be consumed within 8 hours before the bath). This bath is supposed to help detoxify the body. Check with your doctor if you are pregnant before taking this bath.

See Flu Fighter recipe in the next chapter. Also, see olive leaf extract benefits in Chapter 7 under Fungal Infections and Candida.

Hosea 4:6
"My people perish for lack of knowledge…"

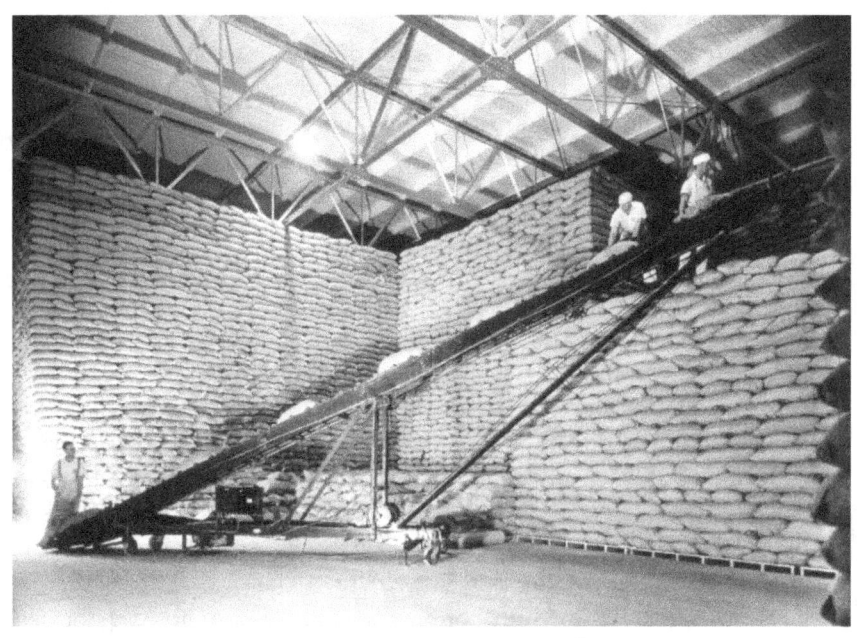

Workers stack bags of white satin sugar in a warehouse.
Reportedly, cancer feeds off of sugar.

Chapter 6
Flu Prevention

When flu season hits, be sure to wash your hands a lot and use winter gloves when getting groceries or gas. You can stock up on at least two weeks worth of groceries so you only have to go to the store twice a month to limit your exposure to germs. The television show "MythBusters" found that a sneeze can travel up to thirty-nine miles per hour and travel up to twenty feet.

Don't touch your head with unwashed hands, especially your eyes, nose, mouth, and ears. Sometimes putting hand lotion on your hands helps you from touching your eyes. Use tissues if you need to touch your eyes.

Get plenty of sleep, be physically active, manage stress, drink plenty of fluids, and eat nutritious food. Avoid close contact with sick people.

Take the time to get the flu vaccine in the fall. Talk to your doctor about when to vaccinate your children. Some children, depending on their age, may require more than one shot. Also, if you get the flu, talk to your doctor about antiviral drugs; which can make the illness milder and shorten the duration of the illness. These drugs must be administered within two days of getting ill so timing is important.

The elderberry juice/extract was used at the Panama Canal to treat a flu epidemic in 1995. Elderberry is used for its antioxidant benefits as well as to lower cholesterol, improve your sight, boost your immune system, help eliminate coughs, colds, flu, bacterial and viral infections, and tonsillitis. If the flu is spreading in your area, start drinking the recommended dosage on the bottle of elderberry juice or extract. It has been found to help build your immune system. It may not completely prevent you from getting the flu but rather shorten the duration of the flu if you do get sick. Many people in the Canal Zone were sick for twelve days and only one was sick for one day because of ingesting elderberry juice. I think there are a lot of factors here. How well-rested are you? What kind of food are you eating? Does the food you eat have any nutrition in it at all?

Most elderberries are edible when picked ripe and then cooked. However, some genus can be poisonous if not cooked. It is recommended for safety reasons to always cook the berries to enhance their taste and digestibility and to avoid getting sick. You can purchase elderberry jam, wine, juice, extract, pills, and lozenges to boost your immune system. It is also noted that elderberries may help reduce cancer, asthma, bronchitis, infection of the urinary tract, and bladder inflammation.

Ground ginger (five to six dashes) in a drink (tea, water, or diet ginger ale) helps alleviate a sore throat. Garlic is also an antiviral and antifungal vegetable. Zinc kills replication of viruses, and the flu is considered a virus.

A scientist in Spain proved that honey contains a natural ingredient that kills influenza germs and helps protect people from the flu. There are many fake honey sellers out there so make sure you know your honey's origin.

Yogurt with ten grams of sugar or less per serving is a great flu-fighting food that boosts your immunity. You can make a smoothie with a probiotic dairy product called kefir. You can purchase a culture starter kit and make your own yogurt at home. All you do is add the kefir grains (culture starter) to milk and let it culture at room temperature for one to two days. That's it! Kefir has more probiotics than store-bought yogurt. You can buy kefir at most health food stores and at the Cultures for Life website.

Flu Buster Soup

1 tablespoon olive oil
1/2 small yellow onion, chopped
2 to 3 cloves garlic, peeled and minced
1/4 teaspoon ground turmeric
1 teaspoon ginger root, peeled and diced
2 small potatoes, peeled and chopped
1/2 head of cauliflower, chopped
1 medium zucchini, chopped
2 large carrots, chopped
4 stalks of celery, chopped
Salt and pepper to taste
Juice of one lemon
4 cups chicken broth
1/2 teaspoon cayenne pepper
Greek yogurt for serving (optional)

Use a large stockpot and heat the olive oil over medium heat. Add the onion, garlic, and turmeric. Sauté until onions are soft. Stir. Add the remaining vegetables. Salt and pepper to taste. Add the juice of the lemon. Stir. Add the broth, cayenne pepper, and season to taste. Cover and bring to a boil for ten minutes or until the vegetables are soft. Blend with an immersion blender until smooth and creamy. A regular blender can be used in smaller portions, if needed. Heat the soup through in the stockpot. Serve with Greek yogurt, if desired.

Flu Fighter Soup

3 cups water
1 cup quinoa, dry
3 tablespoons extra-virgin olive oil
1 big yellow onion, chopped
1/8 teaspoon turmeric powder
5 to 8 cloves garlic, minced
Salt, pepper, and crushed red chili flakes to taste
1 big carrot, finely chopped
5 mushroom caps, finely chopped
1/4 cup coriander, finely chopped
6 cups chicken broth
1 cup kale, chopped

In a saucepan, add three cups water. Bring to boil and add quinoa. Cook for six to nine minutes. Drain. Rinse.

In a skillet, heat oil, sauté the onions, add turmeric, garlic, salt, and red chili flakes. Add carrots, mushrooms, and coriander. Cook for a couple of minutes. Add the quinoa and chicken broth. Heat through until carrots are soft. Add kale, and heat until kale is wilted. Add salt and pepper to taste. It is best to consume this before you get sick, but it will make you feel better if you have the flu.

Green Smoothie Flu Fighter

2 oranges, peeled
1/2 lime, peeled
1 ripe banana
1-inch of ginger root, peeled
1/2 cup parsley
1 cup of kale
1/2 ripe bell pepper
Water for blending

Combine all ingredients in a blender and blend until smooth.

Orange and Coconut Smoothie

1 cup orange juice
1-1/2 cups coconut milk
6 clementine oranges
2 teaspoons raw or dried ginger
2 lemons, juiced
4 tablespoons melted coconut oil
1 cup spinach, tightly packed
1 cup oats (optional)
2 tablespoons chia seeds (optional)
4 tablespoons of raw manuka honey (optional)
20 drops of Echinacea (optional)

Blend the first six ingredients until smooth. Add the spinach and blend again. Add optional ingredients one at a time until smooth. Add water to thin out if needed. Makes two servings. Serve daily for best results.

The following lines repeated from Chapter 5: Cold Prevention.

Foods Rich in Vitamin C

Organic strawberries, oranges, sweet red peppers, broccoli, lemons, lime, and grapefruit all help boost your immune system. This produce is great for your overall health.

Foods Rich in Iron

Lean, grass-raised red meats and poultry and beans provide iron-rich foods that help to fight off infections.

Also, see olive leaf extract benefits in Chapter 7 under Fungal Infections and Candida.

Chapter 7
Other Healthful Tips

Cancer Prevention Strategies
Avoid genetically modified foods. Eat so that your diet consists of at least 50 percent raw foods. If you already struggle with cancer, avoid wheat, gluten, and all forms of sugar. Keep fructose consumption below twenty-five grams per day, and fifteen grams is even better. Less is more.

Eliminate processed foods and junk foods. They don't fuel your body with any nutrition. What happens to your car when you stop putting fuel in it? It stops working, and so does your body when you don't give it anything with nutrition. Processed food and junk food does not give your body any nutrition.

Reduce eating non-organic animal products. Consider an enzyme therapy. Work exercise into your lifestyle. Get outside and get fifteen minutes of sunshine or take a vitamin D supplement. Get at least eight hours of sleep. Reduce the stress in your life by forgetting about the small stuff. Will it really matter in a day, a week, a year? Work on breathing exercises. Turn it into some fun with the kids in your life by blowing bubbles; even in the winter, they will freeze and roll across the ground. Reduce toxins and radiation exposure. Skip those yearly X-rays and go three to five years if there is no imminent need. Learn to love one another, and do something good for someone in need. It will make you feel great!

Also, read about the growth hormone rBGH listed under the acne section below even if you don't have acne.

Top Ten Natural Antibiotics
1. Raw honey—Salve Regina University in Newport, Rhode Island, reaffirmed that raw honey is one of the best natural antibiotics.
2. Colloidal silver—Before 1938, colloidal silver was used by doctors as their main substance to battle bacteria. Colloidal silver promotes healing. I know of one individual who got rid of a throat tumor using this product. They gargled with it and did not drink it.
3. Pascalite—This bentonite clay is found in the mountains of Wyoming. The clay is used topically to draw out infections from wounds in hours or days.
4. Turmeric—Turmeric is a herb used in Chinese medicine to treat infections because it obtains antibacterial and anti-inflammatory qualities. It also has been used topically to treat skin lesions.
5. Oil of oregano—As an essential oil, it has antibacterial, antioxidant, antiseptic, antiviral, antifungal, anti-inflammatory, antiparasitic, and pain-relieving properties. Studies at Georgetown University show that oil of oregano is almost as effective as antibiotics.

6. Tea tree oil—This oil is great for treating skin infections and toenail fungus.
7. Olive leaf extract—An ancient remedy, this extract is being used in European hospitals to fight skin infections.
8. Garlic—Used for thousands of years, it possesses antibiotic, antiviral, and antifungal properties. In the 1700s, it was used to fend off the plague.
9. Echinacea—Currently, it is used to treat colds and the flu. In the past, it was used to treat open wounds, blood poisoning, diphtheria, and other bacteria-related illnesses.
10. Goldenseal—Goldenseal boosts your immune system and is great for respiratory, digestive, and genitourinary tract inflammation. It is a herbal antibiotic.

Inexpensive Cancer Treatments or Alternatives
NOTE: Combining treatments when a tumor is present could result in swelling and be dangerous. You should research these options further before trying them and consult your doctor first. I wanted to mention these options to give you alternatives. There is an abundance of information under each link, and I wanted to make you aware of these options for further research on your own. For more information on alternative treatments refer to these websites and articles:

The Cancer Tutor—Inexpensive (Yet Potent Cancer Treatments)
The Taheebo Tea Club
Essiac Info—The History of Essiac & Nurse Rene M. Caisse
ANH USA—World's Oldest Antibiotic Also Shows Promise as an Anti-
    Cancer Therapy
The Daily Mail Co UK—Silver Bullet for cancer: Metal can kill some
    tumours better than chemotherapy with fewer side effects
The Real Farmacy—The Whole Truth About the Budwig Diet
Budwig Center Natural Therapies—Dr Johanna Budwig Anti-Cancer Diet
    (Budwig Diet: Flaxseed and cottage cheese recipe, plus foods to avoid)
The Healthy Food House—Amazing Herb Kills 98% of Cancer Cells in Just
    16 Hours

Other alternative treatments to research further:
1) Cesium chloride (very alkaline)
2) Baking soda (very alkaline)
3) Calcium (very alkaline)
4) Vitamin C (Don't use potassium ascorbate or limit to 15 percent or less)
    I have found that vitamin C in its natural form is most effective.
    Talk to your doctor about intravenous vitamin C. Also, consume
    it in citrus fruits such as oranges, lemons, and limes.
5) Sister Mary Eymard Poydock, PhD Treatment

6) Honey (see recipe section)

7) DMSO - Chlorine dioxide protocol

8) Robert Barefoot cesium chloride protocol

9) Cell forte IP6

10) Taheebo tea (great when used with essiac tea and ionic silver)

11) Essiac tea (used by a Canadian nurse to cure breast cancer)

12) Ionic silver (colloidal silver—that many have used with great success)

13) Wheatgrass juice protocol

14) Water cure (water and iodized sea salt)

15) Ginger (see recipe section)

16) Vegetable glycern extracted medical cannabinoid tincture

17) Grape seed extract (antibacterial; reportedly outperforms chemotherapy)

18) Sweet wormwood (plant) with iron or artemisia annua Note: Researchers found that when sweet wormwood was mixed with iron, that within one day, 98 percent of the cancer cells were killed. Sources: Natural Society, Healthy Food House, Nation of Change, and Why Don't You Try This websites.

Acne

Avoid wheat and dairy products. Excess growth hormones (rBGH) in dairy products can lead to tumors, cysts, and bacteria that cause acne. Switch dairy milk to almond, cashew, and/or coconut milk. Try adding coconut oil to your diet two to three times a week. Take a new salt shaker that's empty and fill it with aluminum-free baking soda. When you drink your water first thing in the morning, put three dashes of baking soda in the water. The soda kills the bacteria that contribute to acne. You might want to refer to the food charts in Chapter 4 and incorporate more alkaline foods into your diet.

Pimples can be removed from the root by taking three tablespoons of honey and one teaspoon of cinnamon powder paste. Apply this paste on the pimples before sleeping and wash it off the next morning with warm water. Repeat for two weeks.

You might also try bitter apricot kernels, starting with one kernel three times a day with food. This must be taken under adult supervision. Do not take more than directed on the package.

Alzheimer's/Eczema

Coconut oil taken internally will help make your skin softer and lubricate your joints. It also will help the fight against eczema. Eczema can start where there is a patch of dry skin, so if you can keep your skin hydrated and moisturized, eczema can't take hold. Start by consuming one tablespoon of coconut oil a day, especially through the winter season. You also can incorporate avocados into your diet to lubricate your joints internally and also smooth your skin.

I have also found certain acidic foods cause eczema for me. However, when I ate the organic version of the acidic foods, I didn't break out. My thought is that I'm allergic to the pesticides. Also, there has been a rise in pesticide-related childhood diseases.

Coconut oil also can be applied externally to the skin. Prepare a paste with aluminum-free baking soda and coconut oil and apply it to the skin cancer or lesion for at least thirty-eight days. Tape a cotton ball with the baking soda/coconut oil paste on the cancerous legion. Leave it on as long as you can. Reapply as desired throughout the day.

Coconut oil also has been known to help with dementia relief. A doctor married to a man who had dementia tried one shot glass of organic coconut oil a day and found dramatic improvement. Watch Dr. Newport's videos on helping memory loss and Alzheimer's with coconut oil on YouTube.

Applying honey and cinnamon powder in equal parts on the affected parts cures eczema, ringworm, pimples, and all types of skin infections.

Arthritis
Take one cup of hot water and two tablespoons of honey and one small teaspoon of cinnamon powder. Take daily for arthritis pain. Eat before breakfast and, within one week, most people find some relief. Take for a month, and walking pain will greatly diminish.

Asparagus Therapy
In summary of an article originally printed in the *Cancer News Journal*, December 1979, a man with Hodgkin's disease started using asparagus therapy and, in one year, the doctors were unable to find any signs of cancer.

A businessman had bladder cancer for sixteen years and began asparagus therapy and within three months the tumor had disappeared and his kidneys tested normal.

Other stories have been reported of a man with lung cancer, a woman with skin cancer, and many others using asparagus therapy and finding great success. Fresh or canned asparagus can be used. Place the cooked asparagus in a blender and liquefy. Serve four full tablespoons in the morning and another four tablespoons in the evening. It can be taken with hot or cold water. In two to four weeks, patients showed great improvement.

Avoid These Foods
Microwave popcorn contains chemicals that researchers have found to lead to liver and pancreatic cancer, infertility, and tumors.

Non-organic fruits contain pesticides, herbicides, and unsafe fertilizers. The worst on the list are apples, oranges, strawberries, and grapes. Washing the fruit cannot remove the entire residue.

Canned foods are made with a lining in the can called bisphenol-A or BPA, which can lead to infertility, heart disease, and many other illnesses. Canned tomatoes lead the list due to their high acidity levels.

Avoid processed meats such as hot dogs, cold cuts, other meats in a tube, etc., because studies show a strong connection between these foods and colon cancer, rectal cancer, and breast cancer. All processed meats are high in sodium nitrates, chemicals, and preservatives. Stick to three ounces or less of red meat a day and avoid charring it.

Farmed salmon should be avoided due to the unnatural diets they are fed. Also, the farmed salmon can be contaminated with carcinogens, antibiotics, chemicals, and pesticides. Pacific wild caught salmon should be tested for nuclear radiation from Fukushima before consumption. To be safe, test with a Geiger counter.

Potato chips contain unhealthy trans fats, excessive sodium, artificial flavors, preservatives, and artificial colors. A chemical known as acrylamide can be found in potato chips and in cigarettes. The frying at high temperatures causes this chemical in potato chips.

Hydrogenated oils are found in highly processed foods, especially junk foods, and should be avoided.

Pop is loaded with sugar, colorings, and chemicals such as derivative 4-methylimidazole. It takes thirty-two glasses of an alkaline beverage to neutralize twelve ounces of pop, according to the Better Health Thru Research website.

Highly processed white flours raise blood sugar levels and contain a large amount of carbohydrates with a known link to breast cancer.

Genetically modified foods (GMOs) have been modified by chemicals that have been known to cause birth defects and fast-growing tumors. In laboratory research, third-generation mice raised on GMOs were found to be sterile. Almost all grains in the United States have been genetically modified.

Refined sugars provide a quick energy source for cancer cells. Read labels on canned or bottled foods. Remember, four grams of sugar equals one sugar cube. Eliminate as much sugar and sugar derivatives, including fructose and corn syrup, from your diet as possible.

Artificial sweeteners have been found to increase weight gain and make the body crave sweets. Increasing evidence shows that the chemicals used in artificial sweeteners are toxic to the body and can cause cancer and other health problems. Anything consumed and not recognized by the body is turned into fat.

Foods that contain a large amount of salt can cause stomach cancer. Avoid foods that are pickled, smoked, and highly salted. Stick to 1,500 milligrams (about 3/4 teaspoon) of sodium daily for a healthy diet. Research your favorite restaurant meals online and find those meals that are the lowest in sodium. Many fast food meals contain more than three days worth of sodium. Excess sodium also can cause damage to your arteries and veins, which can lead to heart disease.

Bladder Infections

Mix two tablespoons of cinnamon powder and one teaspoon of honey together. Stir into one cup of lukewarm water and drink it. It destroys bladder germs.

Bra Studies and Breast Cancer

Physicians and researchers have found that lymph drainage can be impeded if you wear a tight-fitting bra. Tight-fitting brassieres inhibit the excretion of all the toxins you are exposed to daily, such as aluminum in antiperspirants. The study found that women who wore tight-fitting bras all day (twenty-four hours) had a 75 percent chance of getting breast cancer. Women who wore tight-fitting bras more than twelve hours per day, but not overnight, had a one in seven chance of getting breast cancer, and those who wore a tight-fitting bra less than twelve hours a day had a one in fifty-two chance. Those who very rarely wore bras had a one in one hundred and sixty-eight chance of getting breast cancer. Avoid consuming soda, pop, or caffeinated drinks, which also can affect fertility.

Breast Cancer

Those who have breast cancer must keep their insulin levels within normal ranges. If they do this, they can cut their risk of cancer recurrence in half and cut the risk of death by two-thirds.

Cancer Bush, Suderlandia Fructosate, or Kankerbos

This plant called cancer bush, reportedly works wonders on AIDS patients. It has been used on people who were near death and, after using this plant, the AIDS patient was able to rise up, have energy and appetite, and feel free of depression. In Africa, the plant is used to fight against tuberculosis. Strictly Medicinal Seeds is one website that offers the seeds for planting.

Cholesterol

Take three teaspoons of cinnamon powder and two tablespoons of honey and mix together. Stir into sixteen ounces of tea water. Many people have found a 10 percent reduction in cholesterol levels as soon as two hours.

Deodorant and Antiperspirant

Many products contain toxic aluminum, which is a neurotoxin that is absorbed through the skin, according to the *Journal of Applied Toxicology*. Alternative options are Primal Pit Paste, Young Living, or do-it-yourself deodorant. See the Powerhouse Healthy Recipes in Chapter 9 for homemade deodorant recipes.

Feminine Hygiene Products

Tampons, pads, and feminine wipes often contain harmful chemicals such as chlorine, dioxins, plastics (bisphenol-A and phthalates), synthetic fibers, and petrochemical additives, fragrances, and chemical-based odor neutralizers. Try to choose brands that use non-toxic or natural components such as organic cotton, no plastics, and minimal absorbency volume materials. Recommended brands include Seventh Generation™, Natracare™, and Glad Rags™.

Folic Acid

Folic acid targets cancer cells and is being researched further at Purdue University.

Foods With Vitamin B17

Because vitamin B17 (found in seeds, fruits, nuts, beans, sprouts, leaves, and tubers) tastes bitter, man has crossbred the substance to improve the flavor, thus eliminating a lot of the vitamin B17. This is the missing vitamin in modern man's diet. Sources of vitamin B17 include:

Domestic blackberry, wild blackberry, boysenberry, chokecherry, wild crabapple, market cranberry, Swedish lingonberry, cranberry, currant, elderberry, gooseberry, huckleberry, loganberry, mulberry, quince, and raspberry.

Apple seeds, apricot kernels, buckwheat, cherry seed, flax, millet, nectarine seed, peach seeds, pear seeds, plum seeds, prune seeds, and squash seeds.

Black beans, black-eyed peas, fava, garbanzo, green peas, lentils, and kidney, lima (U.S.), lima (Burma), mung, and shell beans.

Bitter almonds (organic only – others are treated with propylene oxide that can cause cancer), cashew, whole nuts, ground nuts, and macadamia nuts.

Alfalfa, bamboo, fava, garbanzo, lentil, and mung bean sprouts.

Alfalfa leaves, beet tops, eucalyptus, spinach, and watercress leaves.

Cassava, sweet potato, and yam tubers.

Frankincense Essential Oil - A Cancer Kicker

Do not use frankincense if you are pregnant or thinking about becoming pregnant. Consult with your doctor first. Frankincense also can cause blood thinning, gastrointestinal distress, nausea, stomach pain, and hyperacidity. Never use frankincense straight. It needs to be mixed with a carrier oil (another oil).

Take 1/4-cup coconut oil (slightly melted) and place it in a small glass jar. Add to it ten drops of 100 percent pure frankincense essential oil. Stir carefully with a plastic spoon. Apply the ointment to the places on the body that hurt and also to the bottom of the feet. Be sure to have some paper towels on hand to wipe your hands off when done. Place a sealable lid on the jar. Do not consume this mixture. Only certain kinds of frankincense are edible. This is great for managing cancer-related pain and for prostate cancer. Reportedly, frankincense kills cancer cells. You can try this for other cancers as well. The three wise men in the Bible gave the baby Jesus frankincense and myrrh. It is mentioned many, many times in the Bible.

The benefits of frankincense include anti-inflammatory, antitumoral, immune-stimulant, antidepressant and muscle relaxing. It also stimulates the limbic system in the brain and the hypothalamus, pineal, and pituitary glands. It also is antiviral, an antioxidant, antifungal, antibacterial, antiseptic, and an expectorant oil. Its properties are also relaxing and revitalizing.

There is also Neuropathy Rubbing Oil at Walgreens that works well for managing pain. It also helps with managing cancer. It contains ten essential oils, and most of them have anticancer properties. Check their website for availability and location.

Fungal Infections and Candida

Baking soda can be combined with water, oil, or cream and applied to the skin to treat fungal infections. Baking soda is great for treating infections and over-acidity of the mouth. One also can soak in a baking soda bath solution to treat vaginal yeast infections, skin infections, and to draw toxins out of the body.

Raw garlic is a strong proven antifungal. It works well at fighting candida or yeast infections. Grapefruit seed extract kills candida and other microorganisms. Be sure to take a probiotic to replace the good bacteria in your gut. Also, soak in an Epsom salt bath with two cups of warm water for at least twenty minutes.

To defeat candida overgrowth, eliminate processed fast food, refined sugars, carbohydrates, and alcohol. Minimize acid-forming foods (sugars and meats), especially when consumed together at the same meal. Wait at least an hour before consuming sugar after eating red meat. However, sugar should be avoided if you already have a yeast overgrowth problem. Avoid antibiotics if at all possible, steroids, estrogen (birth control pills), and estrogen mimics. Increase raw fruits, vegetables, water, and fiber.

Chopped garlic provides great relief for a cold sore. Leave it on the cold sore for ten minutes and then rinse it off. Repeat if necessary. It may sting a bit, but you will notice quick relief.

Olive leaf extract provides many benefits besides yeast infections. It is available in health food stores in capsules or tablets. Dr. Morton Walker of New

York University and Illinois College of Podiatric Medicine recommends an oleuropein concentration of at least 6%. For preventative measures, it is recommended to use one to two capsules of 250 to 500 milligrams. Caution: Olive leaf extract should not be used with antibiotics or other fungus or mold medicines. The list of benefits includes:

Prevents bacterial, viral, and retroviral infections
Prevention of dental and surgical infections
Aids in relief of HIV, herpes, and shingles
Is an effective treatment for colds, flu, and pneumonia
Aids in relief of chronic fatigue syndrome
Increases blood flow and reduces free radical damage
Helps in alleviating athlete's foot, mycotic nails, yeast infections, and chlamydia

Gloves

In the winter months (or cold and flu season), use gloves when grocery or department store shopping. If you can prevent yourself from touching your eyes, nose, or mouth while in public, you'll be miles ahead.

Grape Seed Extract

Researchers from the University of Colorado Cancer Center reported that grape seed extract targeted and stopped the growth of cancer cells. The more aggressive the cancer cells, the more effective grape seed extract is at targeting and stopping their growth. Grape seed extract also has been studied in its treatment of leukemia, diabetes-related eye disease, loss of vision due to aging, swelling from an injury, and Alzheimer's disease.

Gout

Gout can be caused from a diet rich in acidic foods, which increases the uric acid levels in the body. In other words, stop eating so many sweets, especially right after a protein-rich meal. This leads to arthritis, joint pain, and uric acid crystallization in the joints.

If you make a sugary rich liquid from sugar and water and hang a string in it for a period of time (a couple of weeks), it will grow crystals. The same thing will happen in your joints when you consume too many sugary foods or carbohydrates that break down into sugar (starches, white food like breads, crackers, pastas, etc.).

If you can wait two hours after your meal to consume any sugary food or drinks, this will stop the formation of crystals in the joints, especially in your toe joints. Have you ever seen an innermost toe joint inflamed where the innermost toe is leaning toward the other toes? That is caused by a buildup of crystals in the joint, forcing the toe out of alignment. Gout also can lead to painful kidney stones. Your body is too acidic, which also can make it hard for your body to fight off infections and cancer. Cut back on dairy products as they also can have a lot of sugar in them. Refer back to Chapter 4 and incorporate more foods in the 8.5 to 10-pH range. For an alkalizing drink, see the Ginger-N-Juice Iced Tea and the Berry Fruit Smoothie recipes in Chapter 10.

Hair Care
Many shampoos and conditioners can contain a cancer-causing paraben, synthetic "fragrance" chemicals, sulfates, and other chemicals. Try to find hair care products that do not contain cocamide diethanolamine (cocamide DEA), which is a known carcinogen in the foaming agent and thickener.

Hand and Body Lotions
Avoid lotions that contain diethanolamide (DEA), monoethanolamides (MEA), triethanolamides (TEA), monoisopropanolamides (MIPA), and ethoxylated alkyloamides (PEG). Instead, use pure coconut or jojoba moisturizing oils.

Hand Sanitizer
Hand sanitizers don't work as well as they are cracked up to be because they kill good, protective bacteria as well as the bad bacteria. Many brands contain triclosan, triclocarbon, and synthetic fragrance chemicals, which are absorbed into the skin. A 5 percent vinegar solution in a small spray bottle is a good substitute. It is 99 percent effective and non-toxic. Young Living brand sells an all-natural hand purifier called Thieves, which is made up of essential oils.

Health and Beauty
Fruit and vegetable consumption helps to keep a youthful appearance. Fast food ages you. We have some people in our high school class that look like they are fifteen years older than what they are because they eat highly processed foods as opposed to unprocessed organic foods. Other people eat healthy foods and bicycle a lot and look just like they did on the day of graduation, even though we have been out of school for more than thirty years.

Organic may be expensive but work with what is on sale and stock up. Some is better than none. Go online and check out the story of a Swedish family of five who were not organic food consumers. Scientists tested their urine for a week and then they switched to organic foods for two weeks while they continued testing of their urine daily. On average, the pesticides found in their bodies dropped by a factor of 9.5 when they consumed organic food. The video can be found on YouTube under The Organic Effect. Their story can also be found on treehugger.com. Search for "Swedes show how eating organic eliminates a family's pesticide load."

Put three dashes of aluminum-free baking soda in your drinking water to make your body pH more alkaline. Viruses can't survive in a 8+ pH environment. If your body is too acidic, you can't fight diseases.

There is an enzyme in green vegetables that fights off cancer. Read the article, "Leafy Greens Essential for Immune Regulation and Tumor Resolution" on Dr. Mercola's website. Eating raw green vegetables, promotes oxygen formation in the body. Be sure to add green vegetables to your meals! This is an immunity building must even if you put them in a smoothie!

Healthy oils such as avocado, coconut, olive, cod liver, and sesame oils help with joint maintenance, arthritis prevention, weight loss, soft skin, and heart health. One tablespoon a day is recommended. Don't use the same oil every day. Mix it up and get the benefits from all of the oils.

Heart Health

Be sure to drink a glass of water first thing in the morning. Your blood thickens via evaporation when you're breathing while asleep. Most heart attacks occur in the morning. So it is important to drink water first thing in the morning to thin the blood so the heart doesn't have to work so hard.

Flossing your teeth eliminates harmful bacteria, which, if not removed, can cause gum disease and may be associated with heart attacks. It is believed that the organisms that cause gum disease leave the mouth and infect the heart, contribute to the build-up of fatty deposits in the heart, and weaken the heart by inflammation.

One teaspoon of salt contains twenty-three hundred milligrams of sodium. Many restaurant meals can contain fifty-five hundred milligrams or more of sodium. When you consume that much sodium, it makes the arteries or veins expand to the point they stretch. Once stretched, those stretched areas can accumulate cholesterol. Too much sodium consumption can lead to stomach cancer and high blood pressure, stroke, or heart attack.

The American Heart Association recommends fifteen hundred milligrams of sodium a day (that's no more than 3/4 teaspoon salt). The Heart Association states that the average American and Canadian consumes twice the daily-recommended dosage. While iodized sodium is a necessity, we don't need a lot of it. Bread, processed meats, processed foods, bagged or boxed food, pizza, fast foods, and soups are major sources of sodium overload. Children who eat high amounts of sodium are far more likely to develop high blood pressure as adults.

Consuming large amounts of sodium also will affect your appearance and health by causing extreme thirst, nausea, dizziness, stomach cramps, vomiting, diarrhea, bloating, puffiness, weight gain, dehydration, hypertension (damaging blood vessels), osteoporosis, high blood pressure, stroke, kidney disease or stones, and/or stomach cancer.

Make a paste of honey and cinnamon powder. Use it on your toast for breakfast. It reduces cholesterol and has the potential of saving you from a heart attack. Regular use of cinnamon honey strengthens the heartbeat. Honey and cinnamon revitalize the arteries and veins.

High Triglycerides

One of the main causes of coronary artery disease stems from high fructose corn syrup consumption. By eliminating high fructose corn syrup, aka pop, candy, desserts, some ketchups, some processed foods with high fructose corn syrup, highly refined sugars, and carbohydrates high on the glycemic index, you can drop your triglyceride count. The fructose is dumped into the liver and the liver releases triglycerides in response. Triglyceride medications are designed to work through the liver. So if you can modify your diet, you may not need medication. Check with your doctor before dropping any medications.

Homemade Hair Loss Remedies

Use four drops of rosemary essential oil in one ounce of castor oil. Gently rub on to your scalp and wait twenty minutes. Shampoo it out. Use once or twice a week.

Another remedy is to use two drops of rosemary essential oil and two tablespoons of coconut oil. Apply it to your hair and massage the scalp. Leave in for half an hour and shampoo out. You can use this remedy several times a week.

One remedy is to heat coconut oil with amla (Indian gooseberry) until the amla pieces are charred. Strain and cool the oil. Massage your scalp and leave it on for 30 minutes. Shampoo your hair. Use once a week.

This remedy uses one tablespoon of dried Indian gooseberry powder and one tablespoon of lemon juice. Apply the juice and leave on for twenty minutes before shampooing out. Lemon juice can lighten your hair color over time.

This next remedy uses one part lemon juice and two parts coconut oil. Apply it to your hair and scalp and leave it on for thirty minutes. Shampoo it out. Repeat once or twice a week.

Fenugreek (methi) is effective in treating hair loss. The seeds have hormone antecedents, proteins, and nicotinic acid, great for enhancing hair growth and stimulating hair follicles. Soak one cup of fenugreek seeds in water overnight. The next morning, grind the seeds into a paste. Apply to your hair and cover with a shower cap for forty minutes. Rinse and shampoo your hair. Use this remedy daily for thirty days.

Aloe vera has alkalizing properties that can help bring the scalp and hair's pH to a desirable level, promoting hair growth. Apply aloe vera juice or gel to the scalp and leave it on for a few hours. Shampoo it out with lukewarm water. Use this formula three to four times a week. You also can drink one tablespoon of aloe vera juice daily on an empty stomach.

Take one tablespoon of freshly ground flaxseeds daily with a glass of water in the morning. Ground flaxseeds also can be added to your salads, soups, smoothies, and other dishes. Use flaxseed oil and apply it to your scalp. Leave it on for twenty minutes and shampoo it out.

In general, eating green vegetables, fresh fruits, iron, vitamin A, and Vitamin C help with the problem of hair loss. Eat these foods as much as possible.

Hot Flashes
Try two fish oil capsules with breakfast each day. The fish oil taste will go away after a couple of weeks. Also, apply a cold pack on the back of the neck for a few minutes at the onset of a hot flash.

Infertility
Studies show that too much caffeine (approximately two hundred milligrams) may increase the risk of miscarriage and that one cup of premade coffee (approximately three hundred milligrams) can decrease your chances of conceiving.

The avocado contains most of the thirteen vitamins needed for survival. Having these essential nutrients boosts the chances of fertility. Consuming one avocado a week balances hormones. Eating three avocados a week improves your odds for conceiving. A balanced diet including vegetables and fruits also helps. The ancient Aztecs deemed the avocado the fertility fruit.

Leg Cramps
Leg cramps have many possible causes such as poor blood circulation, overexerting yourself during exercise, especially in the heat, insufficient stretching before exercise, fatigue, lack of fluids, magnesium and/or potassium and/or calcium deficiency, malfunctioning nerves, or a side effect of some prescription drugs.

Many people drink apple cider vinegar or pickle juice for immediate relief and raw garlic or ginger for preventative relief. For immediate relief, try extending your leg straight out and pull the top of your foot back toward your head. You may have to press through it, but it will force the muscle to relax.

Migraines
Migraines can be caused by many factors such as hormonal changes, foods (cheese, salty, processed), food additives, drinks, stress, stimuli, changes in sleep, physical factors, medications, weather changes associated with barometric pressure, medications, and a drop in blood sugar. At the first sign of a migraine, take two spoonfuls of honey and lie down, covering your eyes for thirty to sixty minutes. You also might try adding vitamin B3 to your diet on a regular basis.

Mosquito Repellant
If you are going to be out in a mosquito-laden area, try consuming a couple

of cloves of raw garlic and three to four slices of onions (mostly raw or slightly cooked for best results). You also can cook the garlic and onions with a burger and consume all of it. Your body will exude an odor that the mosquitoes will not like. They may hover near your skin, but they will not land and make a feast out of you. If you find it is not working, eat some more! This will usually last about four to five hours.

Nature's Antibiotic, Colds, Sore Throat, and Coughs

Garlic is nature's antibiotic. A study performed by Washington University found garlic to be one hundred times more effective than the top two most popular antibiotics on the market. Medicinally, garlic has many uses, such as reducing symptoms of colds, coughs, sore throats, and sinus infections. The Amish have been known to swallow small whole cloves to cure a sore throat or oncoming cold. It also can be applied to the skin externally for infections. Garlic also is known to reduce blood sugar and high blood pressure. It helps to boost your immune system. Many say it is also used as a de-wormer, although it should not be used on your pet without first checking with your veterinarian.

When garlic is mixed with raw honey, it becomes an even more potent healer. Chop raw garlic to release allicin—a potent ingredient that helps heal. Then place the chopped garlic in a clean pint jar. Slowly pour raw wildflower honey over the chopped garlic. Stir using a knife or chopstick to get the air bubbles out. Cover and label your jar. Put it in a cupboard for two to four weeks. Use the honey with or without the garlic. The shelf life of garlic honey is three months. Take the mixture by the spoonful, preferably with tea at the first sign of a cough, cold, or sore throat.

At the first sign of a sore throat—that tiny tickle, cough, and throat clearing—take a cup of hot green tea, add honey and six dashes of ground ginger. Drink and enjoy. Within a half an hour, you should find relief. Ground ginger helps with an upset stomach, too. Take one zinc pill with food. Get a good night's sleep.

Overall Good Health

There is a video online about a 110-year-old man in Mesa, Arizona, who is vibrant and healthy. When asked what his secret was, he replied he incorporated five foods into his diet: garlic, honey, cinnamon, chocolate, and olive oil. He also exercised regularly. I remember my grandmother, who lived to be 105, liked honey in the comb. She would pull out a slab from the jar and put it on a plate and cut off a chunk and chew on it. She also ate plenty of mustard potato salad (some mustards have turmeric in them), loved gingersnap cookies (ginger), ate lima beans (vitamin B17), and berries (B17 - especially organic strawberries). She preferred salty foods as opposed to sugary foods.

Sinus Congestion

At the first sign of a sinus headache, take an Advil® Cold & Sinus tablet. Get plenty of rest. Check the moisture content in your home. If it is less than 42 percent, install a humidifier. You can purchase a hygrometer, an instrument used for measuring the moisture content in the atmosphere. Keep the moisture levels at 42 to 50 percent. A sinus rinse bottle is very effective. If you have been in a dusty environment with airborne particulates, use a sinus rinse as soon as possible. Use distilled water and not tap water. Distilled water can be purchased at your local grocery store.

Soaps

Benzyl acetate is a perfume chemical linked to adenomas, carcinomas, stomach tumors, and pancreatic cancer. Recommended soaps are Dr. Bronner's Pure-Castile Liquid Soap and bar soaps, Nubian Heritage, and One with Nature.

Sunscreen

Sunscreen products have been known to contain harmful additives such as oxybenzone, avobenzone, octisalate, octocrylene, homosalata, and octinoxate. Many products contain retinyl palmitate, a type of vitamin A that can actually increase your risk of skin cancer when exposed to the sun. Cover up with long sleeves, a wide-brimmed hat, and long pants if you are going to be out in the sun for a long period of time. Other recommended brands are Dr. Mercola's Natural Sunscreen Lotion, Badger Natural & Organic Sunscreens, and Aubrey Organics.

Toothpaste

See Tom's Toothpaste recipe in the Powerhouse Healthy Recipes in Chapter 9. Commercially made toothpaste can contain toxic additives such as fluoride, propylene glycol, triclosan, and plastics. The Harvard School of Public Health has performed many studies on this subject. There is also a study published in the journal *Langmuir*. Stick to natural toothpaste products such as Dr. Bronner's All-One Toothpaste, Auromere Ayurvedic Toothpaste, Tom's of Maine Natural Toothpaste, Spry Dental Defense Toothpaste, Desert Essence Toothpaste, Jason Toothpaste, Nature's Answer PerioBrite Natural Toothpaste, or make your own.

All-Purpose Cleaning Product

1/2 cup vinegar
1/4 cup aluminum-free baking soda
2 quarts water
2 tablespoons lemon juice

Add together and stir well. Place in an empty spray bottle. Label the bottle.

Stain Remover

2 parts hydrogen peroxide
1 part Dawn™ dish soap

Combine the peroxide and soap. Mix. Place in a spray bottle. Spray on stains. Leave for 30 minutes. Rinse. Plain hydrogen peroxide is also great for spraying on mold. Black mold can cause cancer so use protective clothing and a mask when dealing with black mold or hire a professional.

Dog and Cat Cancer Prevention Tips

For preventing cancer in dogs and cats, you might consider having your pet spayed or neutered at a young age. Breast cancer in females and testicular cancer in males can be prevented by doing this. Many specialists suggest adding vitamins C and E to your pet's diet for prevention, and others suggest a certain type of diet or food or the omission of certain foods in their diet.

An anti-inflammatory and anticancer dog diet consists of real whole foods, preferably raw. High-quality protein, muscle meat, organs, and large bones are good except small pieces of bone can be chewed off and lodged in organs—so watch your pet carefully! Include moderate amounts of animal fats and high levels of EPA and DHA (omega-3 fatty acids), fresh-cut veggies, and a bit of fruit (except apples or fruits with similar type seeds). No grains or starches are recommended. A vitamin/mineral supplement and a few probiotics, digestive enzymes, and super green foods are suggested. Consult your veterinarian for the best plan of action.

Reduce your pet's exposure to toxins such as chemical pesticides like flea and tick preventatives, lawn chemicals, weed killers, herbicides, tobacco smoke, flame-retardants, detergents, soaps, cleansers, dryer sheets, and room deodorizers.

The leading cause of death in dogs over the age of ten is cancer, but if caught early, it can be curable. Certain types of dog breeds are more susceptible to cancer, such as Golden Retrievers, Bernese mountain, boxers, and flat-coated retrievers. Mixed breeds come from a larger gene pool and are much less likely to get genetic-based cancers.

Good oral hygiene for your pet can help decrease oral cancers.

Access to fresh green grass that hasn't been sprayed with chemicals is helpful for your cat or dog. Grass plants are high in cancer-fighting nitrolosides. This is why you see dogs and cats occasionally chewing on grass when they don't feel well.

You might want to consider a home remedy for fleas on your furry feline or dog. There are natural flea treatment remedies to check out on the Easy-Home-Made and the Knowledge Weighs Nothing websites.

Foods Hazardous to Dogs

Most dogs like to be with us and eat what we eat. However, there are certain foods that are hazardous to your furry friend(s). Consult your veterinarian immediately if your dog has consumed any of these foods.

Hazardous foods for canines:
Avocado
Raw bread dough
Chocolate
Ethanol (also known as ethyl alcohol, grain alcohol, or drinking alcohol)
Grapes
Raisins
Hops
Macadamia nuts
Moldy foods
Onions and garlic
Xylitol (non-caloric sweetener found in sugar-free gum and baked goods)

Chapter 8
Beneficial Alkaline Foods

Leafy greens may not be your cup of tea, but there are some very important reasons to include them in your diet on a regular basis. First of all, leafy green vegetables include an enzyme that helps resolve cancerous lesions. My friend's parents both came down with cancer at the same time. When my friend asked the doctor why that might be, he responded, "They were not getting an enzyme that they needed in their diet found in green vegetables." When we helped my friend clean her parents' house, we found a TV dinner reheated and stuck to the burner on the stove. No greens in sight.

The green vegetables help to make your body pH more alkaline, an environment where viruses have a hard time surviving. So, throw a couple of leafy greens on your sandwich, add a small salad to your meal, or make a meal out of a salad with all of your favorite toppings, using other alkaline vegetables like cucumbers, red peppers, broccoli, celery, and avocado slices. Also check out smoothie recipes with greens in Chapter 9. Vegetables are not very high in calories, so they should make the bulk of your diet by volume.

Immunity lies in the lining of your digestive system where cells protect the body from "bad" bacteria. These cells play a factor in food allergies, inflammation, preventing weight gain, and bowel cancers.

When ingesting leafy green vegetables, your body produces a hormone that helps protect it from pathogenic bacteria and that promotes beneficial bacteria, resolves cancerous lesions, and heals small wounds and abrasions in the gut.

See the baking soda and molasses remedy at the Earth Clinic website.

Lemon a Day Keeps Cancer Away
Cut two to three slices of lemon and place it in a cup. Add drinking water; which will become alkaline water. Drink it for a whole day.

Lemon (or citrus) is a miraculous product to kill cancer cells. It is 10,000 times stronger than some conventional cancer treatments. Try eating the fruit in different ways such as making a pulp out of it or juicing it; prepare drinks, sorbets, pastries, etc. If you are using lemons or other citrus to fight cancer, eat it without sugar because cancer feeds off of sugar.

Laboratory tests reveal that lemon destroys malignant cells in twelve cancers, including colon, breast, prostate, lung, and pancreatic. Lemon extract destroys malignant cancer cells, and it does not affect healthy cells.

Chapter 9
Powerhouse Healthy Recipes

These recipes are not designed to cure cancer but rather to incorporate foods that help to prevent cancer and help to keep cancer at bay. Most of these recipes have been chosen with food items that nourish, help in the fight against cancer, and make the body pH more alkaline. You can prove this to yourself by testing your body pH in the morning by testing your urine with pH test strips (available for purchase online). Urine is more reliable than saliva testing.

It is strongly suggested that you use organic products whenever possible. There was a study done by Dr. Konstantin Korotkov of St. Petersburg, Russia, who found the bio-electrographic glow of organic plants was much brighter and stronger than that of non-organic plants. Sick plants had an uneven, restricted glow. Mature, healthy plants had a strong energy flow. That energy transfers to us if we eat the healthy plants, and it makes us healthy in return.

For the recipes in this chapter, use raw honey and Ceylon cinnamon for best results. If you already have cancer, avoid recipes with sugar. If you find that cooking takes too much energy when you are sick, take a look at the Powerhouse Cancer Fighting Foods listed in Chapter 10 and incorporate as many of them as you can into your diet. You also can choose the simpler recipes. Order from the bulk food organic suppliers listed in Chapter 9, and you can have bulk foods shipped directly to your home.

If you are allergic to certain foods, try the organic version. Many people are allergic to pesticides.

Note: Metric conversion charts can be found on page 106.

Beverages

Cancer Kicker

1/2 lime
1-1/2 cups pineapple
1/4 bunch cilantro
6 leaves romaine lettuce

Put lime and pineapple in a juicer. Add cilantro and romaine. Alternate the ingredients to keep them moving through the juicer. Citrus is great at kicking cancer. This is a great detoxification drink.

Chocolate Dream

1 cup unsweetened vanilla almond milk
3/4 banana, frozen
1 handful kale
1/3 avocado, peeled and pitted
1 tablespoon unsweetened cocoa powder

Add almond milk in blender. Add banana, blend. Add remaining ingredients. Blend until desired thickness. Healthy fats keep you feeling full and keep blood sugar levels stable. Note: The banana doesn't have to be frozen. But freezing bananas that are about to go bad is a good way to "save" them for later use.

Deb's Dandelion Root Tea
(Reportedly kills all kinds of cancer cells)

1 fresh dandelion root
Ground ginger
Aluminum-free baking soda
1 cup water

Note: Talk to your physician about possible interactions with prescriptions or existing conditions. People with blocked bile ducts or gall bladder issues may need to avoid the herb.

Dig up one dandelion root from an area that has not been sprayed. Wash the root (a vegetable brush works well). Chop enough root to make two tablespoons. Pour water in your pan, add the chopped dandelion root, and boil for one minute. Turn off the heat. Steep the liquid for forty minutes. Drink two glasses daily. Drink it warm or cool. This will reportedly make cancer cells commit suicide. To make it more potent, add five to six dashes of ginger and three dashes of aluminum-free baking soda.

For more information watch on YouTube "How to make cancer killing dandelion root tea."

Detoxification Mint Water
(Alkaline Drink)

1 quart water
1 lemon, sliced
1 cucumber, sliced
10 to 12 mint leaves

Mix all ingredients in a pitcher. Place in the refrigerator overnight to infuse. Drink in the morning first thing. All ingredients help to make your body pH alkaline. This drink is great for your overall health.

Diana's Detoxification Drink

4 cups packed leafy greens (kale, variety of lettuce)
1/2 cup almond butter
2 tablespoons hempseeds or ground flaxseeds
3 to 6 medium pitted dates (optional)
1 to 2 medium bananas, frozen and broken into pieces
1 cup ice
2 cups unsweetened chocolate plant-based milk

Blend all ingredients for one minute until smooth and creamy. Makes two servings. Note: The banana doesn't have to be frozen. But freezing bananas that are about to go bad is a good way to "save" them for later use.

Energy Booster

2 to 3 pieces watermelon, about 6 inches long
2 pieces pineapple, about 6 inches long
1 beet, peeled and cut into chunks
1 handful fresh spinach
3 to 4 broccoli florets

Blend all ingredients until smooth. Serve over ice.

Ginger and Citrus Tea Immune Booster
This tea is great for allergies, colds, headaches, indigestion, muscle pain, and joint pain. You can use whichever tea best suits you. Many people prefer a tea like chamomile.

5 cups water
1 lemon, sliced
1 tangerine, sliced
1 tablespoon apple cider vinegar
2 tablespoon cinnamon or 2 cinnamon sticks
Dash of nutmeg
Fresh ginger, peeled and sliced
4 bags of herbal tea

Place all of the ingredients into a saucepan and bring to a simmer. Simmer for two to three minutes. Use honey as a sweetener. For optional sweeteners, add a little milk or flavored creamer.

Ginger Bug
(Recipe uses sugar; do not make if you already have cancer.)

2 cups filtered water
3 grated teaspoons ginger
1/4 cup organic sugar

Add all ingredients to a Mason jar and mix. Cover with cheesecloth or a coffee filter. Each day for five days, stir in 1 tablespoon of sugar and 1 tablespoon grated ginger. Once mixture is active, it will bubble. (If it hasn't become active in eight days, discard and start again.) Keep cultures away from other cultures like Kombucha. Now you can add this to other liquids such as a club soda to make your own sodas. Note: To keep culture alive, keep feeding it sugar and ginger. Reprinted with permission from www.earthiemama.com.

Ginger-N-Juice Iced Tea
(Alkaline Drink)

Organic ginger tea
Purified and alkaline water
1 to 2 tablespoons fresh lemon or lime juice
1/4 cup organic grapefruit juice

Heat the purified alkaline water. Add the ginger tea. Let tea mixture sit for five minutes or until the desired darkness is reached. Let cool. Add citrus juice. Add ice and enjoy! Note: You can heat this during the winter.

Ginger Root Tea

1-inch piece ginger root
1-1/2 cups boiling water

Boil water. Remove from heat and immediately add ginger root. Steep for fifteen minutes. Drink hot or cold.

Healthy Green Juice

1 large handful kale, chopped
1 large handful spinach
1 large beet, quartered
1 cup carrots, sliced (skip the carrots if you already have cancer)
1 cup celery, sliced
1/2 small cucumber, peeled
1 sprig parsley
1 large handful Swiss chard, chopped
3 teaspoons turmeric (optional, great for kicking cancer)
1/8 teaspoon ground black pepper (optional, great for kicking cancer)
1 clove raw garlic (optional, great for kicking cancer)

Blend until smooth in a blender. Pour into a glass and enjoy! Note: Carrots may spike your insulin, and cancer thrives on sugar.

Heart Healthy Cleanser

16 ounces organic raw wheat germ
15 lemons (make sure organic because peelings will be used)
12 cloves garlic
16 ounces organic walnuts
2 pounds raw organic honey

This recipe is an excellent cleanser for the veins, helps the heart, washes the liver, calms the mind, and helps to treat malignancy.

Place the raw wheat in a glass jar. Top it off with water and let it sit for half a day. Cover with gauze. After twelve hours, strain the liquid through the gauze and rinse the wheat. After twenty-four hours, sprouts appear.

In a food processor, add garlic, walnuts, and wheat sprouts. Add five whole lemons (with peel) to the mixture. Juice the remaining lemons and add to the mixture. Add the honey. Stir and store in glass jugs and refrigerate for three days. Take one to two tablespoons thirty minutes before every meal three times a day. If you are treating a tumor, consume a spoonful every two hours.

Homemade Ginger Ale

8 cups of filtered water
2-inch piece of ginger root, minced
1/2 cup organic sugar (Do not use sugar if you already have cancer.)
1/2 teaspoon Himalayan salt
1/2 cup fresh lemon juice
1/2 cup Ginger Bug (see Ginger Bug recipe)

Put three cups of water, minced ginger, sugar, and salt in a pan and bring to a boil. Reduce heat and simmer for five minutes or until sugar is dissolved and it starts to smell like ginger. Remove from heat. Add five cups of water. Once cooled completely, add lemon juice and Ginger Bug recipe and mix. Pour liquid into a two-quart Mason jar or any jars that seal tightly. Leave on counter for two to three days until carbonated. Strain and put in bottles for refrigeration. This recipe reprinted with permission from www.earthiemama.com.

Marvel Magic Juice

2 large beets, peeled
4 long carrots, cleaned
2 apples (any kind)
6 stalks celery
2 limes, peeled
2-inch piece of ginger

Juice the ingredients. Stir and drink. This juice is beneficial for preventing cancer and beating it down. It works great for healing organs and ulcers. It improves airways, lungs, blood pressure, prevent heart attacks, strengthens the immune system, eliminates muscle pain, rehydrates dry eyes, eliminates constipation or diarrhea, eliminates acne, improves bad breath and reduces allergies and hay fever.

Master Tonic
(Antiviral, antibacterial, antifungal, and antiparasitic)

1 (32-ounce) bottle organic apple cider vinegar
1/4 cup chopped garlic
1/4 cup onions
1 habanero pepper (or hottest peppers you can find)
1/4 cup grated ginger
2 tablespoons grated horseradish
2 tablespoons turmeric or 2 turmeric root chunks

It is a good idea to wear gloves and goggles when handling hot peppers. It is difficult to get the heat off of your hands! Warning: Habanero peppers are the hottest peppers on the planet. Blend all ingredients together for a couple of minutes. Strain. Pour liquid back into empty vinegar bottle. Alternative method: Chop all of the ingredients and put in a jar. Pour apple cider vinegar over vegetables until all ingredients are submerged. Leave it in a dark place until the full moon or as long as you want. The longer it sits, the more potent it gets. Strain and bottle the contents. No need to keep in the refrigerator. You also can use it mixed with olive oil for a salad dressing. For sore throat, gargle a bit in the mouth and swallow. For an illness, such as a cold or flu, take about two droppers full or a tablespoon every couple of hours. For daily immune support, drink two droppers full or one tablespoon every day. Build up tolerance to where you can drink a shot glass full of the mixture. Eat an orange, lemon, or lime slice afterward to ease the heat. This recipe reprinted with permission from www.earthiemama.com. You also can buy a bottle at the same website: http://www.earthiemama.com/store/p15/Master_Tonic.html

The Beauty Queen

Juice from 1 lime
1 apple, diced
1 handful spinach
2 kiwi, peeled and diced
1 stalk celery
1 teaspoon honey
Ice

Place ingredients in a blender, blend, and enjoy! The first three ingredients boost the body's immune system, flush out toxins, and reduce inflammation. The kiwi and celery fight free radicals. This is a great detoxification drink.

The Beauty Sheen

10 spinach leaves
1 stalk celery
1/2 cucumber
1/2 cup parsley

Juice all ingredients. Add ice, if desired. Parsley acts as a diuretic to help with bloat. Spinach contains glycoglycerolipids that contain anticancer properties. This drink is rich in vitamins A and C promoting skin health. This is a great detoxification drink.

Tropical Delight

1-1/2 cups unsweetened coconut water
1 cup frozen mango chunks
1 cup frozen pineapple chunks
1 cup leafy greens (baby spinach, kale, or collard greens)
1/4 cup lime juice
1/4 teaspoon cayenne pepper (optional)

Combine all ingredients in a blender and blend until smooth. By combining the vitamin C-rich pineapple and lime juice with the spinach, it helps to enhance the absorption of iron from the leafy greens. Makes two servings.

Tumor Tackler

14 ounces wheat germ
Water
12 cloves garlic
14 ounces walnuts
15 organic lemons (clean skin; do not peel)
2 pounds raw organic honey

Place the wheat germ in a glass jug. Fill the jug with water, cover jug with gauze, and let sit for twelve hours. When the time is up, strain the mixture through the gauze and wash the wheat. After twenty-four hours, sprouts will appear about one to two millimeters long.

In a meat-mincing machine, mix together the garlic, walnuts, and wheat sprouts. Add five whole lemons. Add the juice from ten lemons to the mixture. Add the honey. Stir well. Pour the mixture into glass jug(s) and refrigerate for three days before use.

This recipe helps treat the whole body and many illnesses! To consume it, take one to two tablespoons thirty minutes before every meal (three times a day). For use in eliminating a tumor, take a spoonful every two hours.

Turmeric-Ginger Tea

1 cup water
1/4 teaspoon ground turmeric
1/4 teaspoon ground ginger
2 teaspoons milk, soy milk, or your favorite unsweetened nut milk
Honey or maple syrup, to taste

Bring water to boil in a small saucepan. Add the next two ingredients, reduce heat and simmer for ten minutes. Add milk and stir. Strain tea into a cup and add sweetener to taste.

Turmeric Milk

1 cup whole organic milk
1/4 teaspoon ground or 1/2 teaspoon fresh grated turmeric
1 cardamom, crushed
2 tablespoons almond slivers
Honey, to taste

Combine first four ingredients in a small pan. Bring to a boil and simmer for three minutes. Cool slightly. Add honey to taste.

Turmeric Tea
(Great for tension headaches and muscle/joint pain)

4 cups of water
2 tablespoons grated fresh turmeric root OR
1 heaping teaspoon ground turmeric
5 dashes of ground ginger
Honey/fresh lemon to taste

Boil the water. Add the turmeric. For fresh turmeric, boil the mixture for fifteen to twenty minutes. For powdered turmeric, only boil for ten minutes.

Strain the tea through a fine sieve. Add the ground ginger, honey, and lemon to taste. Stir and serve.

Desserts

Banana Cherry Soft Serve

2 frozen ripe bananas
1-1/2 cups unsweetened cherries, pitted and frozen, divided
2 tablespoons unsweetened coconut milk
1/4 cup dark chocolate chips (70 percent or more cocoa)

Blend bananas, one cup of cherries, and milk until slightly blended. Add more milk if needed. Add remaining cherries and chocolate chips. Blend only a little bit. Serve immediately.

Banana Chocolate Ice Cream

1/2 cup unsweetened cashew milk
1/2 frozen ripe banana
1/4 tablespoon cocoa powder
1/4 teaspoon liquid Stevia (optional)
3 dashes ground cinnamon

You can use a blender or hand blender with a small bowl. Pour milk in blender or bowl. Add frozen bananas. Blend. Add remaining ingredients and blend well. Enjoy!

Chia Pudding

2 tablespoons chia seeds
1/2 cup unsweetened cashew or almond milk
1/4 teaspoon lemon zest
1/2 cup fresh raspberries or strawberries

Pour chia seeds in a small bowl. Add the milk and zest. Add the fresh fruit and mash or blend with hand blender. Cover the bowl and store the mixture in the refrigerator for at least two hours or overnight. Top with more fresh fruit if desired and serve.

Delicious Apricot Truffles

1 cup dried apricots
1 cup dried unsweetened cranberries
1 teaspoon organic orange zest (scrapings of an orange peeling)
2 cups dark chocolate (73 percent cocoa)

Place fruits and zest in a food processor. Process with short pulses until the fruit forms a large ball. Line baking sheet with parchment paper. Form 1-inch balls and place on parchment paper. Melt the chocolate in a double boiler or saucepan over low heat. Dip the balls into the chocolate with a fork and place on the parchment paper. Allow chocolate to harden. Refrigerate if needed. Makes 24 servings.

Guilt-free Cookies

1 egg
2 heaping tablespoons natural peanut butter
4 ripe bananas, peeled
2 tablespoons cocoa powder
1/2 teaspoon aluminum-free baking soda
1/2 cup flour
2 cups quick oats
1 cup dark chocolate chips (optional)

Mix first three ingredients well until creamy, then add the cocoa powder, soda, and flour. Mix well. Add oats, then chocolate chips and mix well. Spoon dough out on baking sheet lined with parchment paper. A small ice cream scoop works well. These cookies do not spread out so you can fit more on the sheet. Bake at 350 degrees Fahrenheit for fifteen minutes.

Heavenly Parfait

Chocolate Pudding Mixture:
1 avocado, cored
1/4 cup raw cacao powder
1/4 cup honey
3 tablespoons unsweetened coconut milk
Dash of salt

Peanut Butter Pudding Mixture:
1/2 cup fresh ground peanut butter (raw is best)
3 tablespoons honey
1/3 cup unsweetened coconut milk, plus a little extra

Blend the avocado, cacao powder, honey, milk, and salt in a food processor until creamy. Pour into a bowl. Clean out the food processor. Blend the peanut butter, honey, and coconut milk (minus the extra milk) in the food processor. If the pudding is too thick, add the extra milk and blend again. Layer the two mixtures in two stemmed glasses. Makes two small servings. Refrigerate leftovers.

Soft Date Cookies

1/3 cup packed chopped raisins
1/3 cup packed chopped dates
1/2 cup mashed bananas
1/4 cup creamy peanut butter
1/4 cup water
1 egg, beaten
1 teaspoon vanilla extract
1 cup quick-cooking rolled oats
1/2 cup all-purpose flour
1 teaspoon aluminum-free baking soda

Preheat the oven to 350 degrees. In a bowl, mix well the first seven ingredients. Next, add remaining ingredients and blend well.

Drop by spoonfuls onto baking sheet with parchment paper or lightly greased sheet. Flatten with a fork. Bake ten minutes or until lightly browned. Cool completely on wire rack. Store in sealed container.

Raisin Oatmeal Guilt-free Cookies

3 mashed ripe bananas
1/3 cup applesauce
1/4 cup almond milk
1 teaspoon vanilla
1 teaspoon cinnamon
2 cups quick oats
1/2 cup raisins (optional)

Mix first five ingredients together. Add oats, then raisins. Mix well. Spoon the dough onto baking sheet with parchment paper. Bake at 350 degrees for fifteen to twenty minutes.

Main Dishes

Banana Almond Pancakes

2 ripe bananas
1 egg
2 heaping tablespoons almond butter
Butter or olive oil for frying
Your favorite berries

Mash the bananas with a fork. Add the beaten egg and stir well. Add the almond butter. Mix well. Melt butter in frying pan. Pour batter into small cakes. Flip pancake occasionally. Serve warm with your favorite berries on top.

Baked Chicken

9 chicken breasts
Olive oil
Onion powder
Dash chili powder
Salt and pepper to taste
Favorite green vegetable
Small salad
Red potatoes, cooked

Place nine fresh chicken breasts on a baking sheet with parchment paper.

Brush with olive oil. Sprinkle with onion powder, chili powder, salt, and pepper to taste. Bake at 350 for twenty minutes or until no longer pink. Store leftovers in the freezer for an easy partial meal. Add vegetables, small salad, and/or a boiled red potato. Red potatoes contain fewer carbohydrates. This recipe works well with fish or poultry.

Cancer Kicking Salad

1 large handful kale, chopped
1 large handful spinach, chopped
1 large handful baby romaine, chopped
1 large handful arugula, chopped
Baby bella mushrooms, sliced
1 small red onion, chopped
1/4 to 1/2 cup zucchini, chopped
1/4 to 1/2 cup squash, chopped
1 small to medium green bell pepper
1/4 to 1/2 cup broccoli, chopped
1/2 cup celery, chopped
1/2 cup red cabbage, chopped
1/2 avocado or 6 tablespoons avocado, cubed
Alfalfa sprouts
Sunflower seeds
Almonds, chopped
Sprouted garbanzo beans
Sprouted mung beans
Sprouted red or green lentils
Bubbies sauerkraut (with only cabbage, water, and salt)

If you can't find all of these ingredients, use what you can find because they are all helpful in the fight against cancer. Prepare ingredients and start with the first four ingredients on a plate. Add remaining ingredients. Use Cancer Kicking Salad Dressing. Makes four small servings or two large servings.

Cancer Kicking Salad Dressing

Cold-pressed extra virgin olive oil
Apple cider vinegar
Dash of oregano
Dash of garlic powder
Dash of turmeric or curry powder
Dash of cayenne pepper

Mix the first two ingredients in a glass jar. Stir well. Pour on the salad. Sprinkle the spices onto the salad. Enjoy!

Broccoli and Kale Soup

2 tablespoons extra-virgin olive oil
8 cups yeast-free, gluten-free vegetable broth
1 head broccoli, cut into small pieces
4 celery stalks
2 handfuls kale
2 handfuls spinach
2/3 cup tahini (sauce made from sesame seeds)
2 teaspoons Celtic sea salt

Place oil and broth in a large stockpot. Bring to a boil, and then add the broccoli. Cover pot and bring to a low rolling boil until broccoli is bright green. Add celery and kale. Simmer until kale is wilted. Remove pot from the heat. Add remaining ingredients. Let cool for fifteen minutes then blend ingredients until smooth.

Chicken Bowl

4 ounces grilled chicken cubes
Snow peas
Broccoli, chopped or cut into small pieces
Mushrooms, sliced (baby bella work well)
Green onions, diced
2 tablespoons low-sodium soy sauce
Cauliflower rice (See Mexican Fiesta Fix (page 66) for cauliflower rice recipe)

Mix ingredients together and serve in a bowl. Enjoy!

Chef Salad

Kale
Mixed lettuce
4 hard-boiled eggs, sliced
Red peppers, sliced
Cabbage, sliced
Celery, sliced
Sliced ham without preservatives (optional)
Portabella mushrooms, sliced (optional)
Low-fat cheese, (optional)
Beet, chopped (optional)
Organic ranch dressing or Olive oil and apple cider vinegar dressing

Place kale and lettuce on dinner plate. Add other desired ingredients and top with your favorite dressing.

Diana's Pizza

1 head cauliflower
2 eggs
1/4 teaspoon salt
1 teaspoon Italian seasoning
1/2 cup mozzarella cheese
Pesto sauce, Alfredo sauce, or pizza sauce (Pizza sauce recipe below)
Green peppers
Onions
Garlic
Mushrooms (baby bella, sliced, or any kind)
Spinach

Cut up cauliflower and run through food processor until rice-sized. Microwave the cauliflower rice for approximately eight minutes. Place on paper towels to drain while cooling. In large bowl, blend two eggs, salt, Italian seasoning, and mozzarella cheese. Add cauliflower rice and mix well. Line a cookie sheet with parchment paper. Place mixture on cookie sheet and flatten to half-inch thick. Bake at 450 degrees for fifteen minutes or golden brown. Take crust out of oven and cover with sauce of choice. Add other toppings. Place back in oven under broiler for five minutes. Bake until slightly brown. Serve warm.

Pizza Sauce

1 (15-ounce) can tomato sauce
1 (6-ounce) can tomato paste
1 tablespoon oregano
1-1/2 teaspoons dried minced garlic
1 teaspoon ground paprika

Mix sauce and paste together. Stir. Add remaining ingredients. Stir.

Eggselent Egg Bites
(Quick breakfast or snack)

1 1/4 cups fresh baby spinach, cooked
4 large eggs
4 egg whites
1 medium sweet onion, diced
2 tablespoons finely chopped fresh parsley
2 tablespoons chia seeds
1/4 teaspoon salt
1/4 teaspoon freshly ground pepper

Preheat oven to 350 degrees. In a medium bowl, beat eggs and egg whites. Add remaining ingredients and mix well. Line muffin tin with foil cupcake liners. Fill cups 2/3 full with egg mixture. Bake for thirty minutes or until set. Remove from oven and let cool. Serve warm or refrigerate.

Grandma's Chicken Soup

8 to 10 cups chicken broth
4 chicken breasts
2 to 3 tablespoons olive oil
Salt and pepper to taste
1 large yellow onion, sliced
2 sweet potatoes, cubed
2 large parsnips, sliced
1 small package baby carrots, sliced
6 stalks celery, sliced
1 small container of mushrooms, sliced
2 stems of parsley

This recipe has been handed down from generations. Pour broth into large stockpot. Place on medium heat. Throw in the peeled and washed vegetables whole if you don't want to take the time the cut them up raw. You can always cut them up when they are cooked and much softer. Food scissors work great for this. Place the chicken breasts on a baking sheet and coat with olive oil. Season with salt and pepper to taste. If the chicken is fresh, bake at 350 degrees for twenty minutes. If the chicken is frozen, bake at 350 degrees for forty minutes or until no longer pink in the center. Slice into small pieces when baked, using food-grade scissors. Place remaining ingredients into stockpot. Boil on medium heat until root vegetables are soft. It takes about 1 1/2 to 2 hours to get to a boiling temperature due to the large size of the recipe. You can make a smaller batch. Season to taste.

Italian Dish

4 ounces ground turkey, cooked
1 tablespoon olive oil
1 small tomato, diced
2 leaves basil, sliced
1 tablespoon garlic, minced
2 tablespoons onion, diced
1 to 2 small zucchinis made into noodles (sliced with julienne peeler)
Salt and pepper to taste

Cook all ingredients together except zucchini noodles. When cooked, pour over noodles. Enjoy!

Lean Greens

2 to 3 tablespoons butter
1 tablespoon water
2 stalks celery, sliced
1 green pepper, diced
3 scallions, chopped (separate whites and greens)
3 ounces green beans, cut
1 head broccoli, chopped
1 large zucchini, sliced
Salt and pepper to taste

In skillet, combine water and butter. Sauté celery, pepper, and white scallion parts until soft. Next, sauté green beans until soft. Add remaining vegetables and cook until tender. Season to taste. Serve.

Mexican Fiesta Fix

4 ounces chicken, cooked and shredded
1 can red kidney beans, drained
1 small tomato, diced
1 small green pepper
1 small onion
1/4 avocado, sliced
2 tablespoons salsa
Cauliflower rice

Mix all ingredients together except cauliflower rice. Serve over cauliflower rice.

To make the cauliflower rice, cut the florets off the head of cauliflower, leaving behind the hard stem. Blend the florets in a food processor. The rice can be bagged and stored in the freezer for later use or cooked in a pan with a tablespoon of olive oil for five to eight minutes until desired tenderness.

Slow Cooker Beef Barley Soup

1-1/2 pounds grass-fed hamburger
3 tablespoons olive oil
1 teaspoon salt
1 teaspoon ground black pepper
2 teaspoons garlic powder
10 cups low sodium beef broth
4 stalks celery, sliced
1 small bag baby carrots, ready-to-eat kind
6 green onions, chopped
1/2 cup chopped fresh parsley
1 cup barley
1 teaspoon dried thyme

Brown hamburger in skillet. Drain grease off into glass jar. Place meat in slow cooker. Add salt, pepper, and garlic powder. Stir. Add broth, celery, carrots, green onions, parsley, and barley. Cover and cook on low setting for six to eight hours until tender. Add thyme before serving.

Spinach Lasagne

2 pounds fresh spinach
4 tablespoons grated Parmesan cheese, divided
1 cup part-skim ricotta cheese
1/4 teaspoon nutmeg
1/4 teaspoon salt
Fresh ground black pepper to taste
1 tablespoon olive oil
2 cloves garlic, crushed
1/2 cup chopped onion
1/2 cup chopped bell pepper
2 cups tomato sauce
1/2 teaspoon basil
1/2 teaspoon oregano
1/2 teaspoon thyme
1/2 pound lasagne noodles

Wash spinach and steam for two minutes. Chop the spinach and add two tablespoons of Parmesan cheese and the ricotta, nutmeg, salt, and pepper.

Sauté in oil the garlic, onion, and bell pepper until wilted. Stir in tomato sauce and remaining seasonings. Cover and simmer until ready to use. Preheat oven to 350 degrees. Cook lasagne noodles according to package instructions. In a 9-by-13-inch baking dish, layer noodles alternating with cheese-spinach mixture and tomato sauce, ending with remaining Parmesan cheese. Bake at 350 degrees for thirty minutes or until bubbly brown.

The Best Antibiotic Soup
(100x stronger than antibiotics)

50 cloves of organic garlic, cleaned, peeled
1/4 cup and 2 tablespoons olive oil, divided
2 tablespoons of butter
2 large red onions, diced
Fresh or dried herbs to taste (thyme, parsley, bay leaves)
6 cups chicken broth
3 cups stale organic bread, cubed or crushed
1 cup sour cream
Salt and pepper

Preheat the oven to 350 degrees. Chop off the ends of the garlic bulbs, spread the cloves on foil and drizzle with 1/4 cup olive oil. Wrap in foil. Place the foil on a cookie sheet and bake for one-and-a-half hours. Cool.

In a large soup pot, mix remaining olive oil and butter over medium heat. Add red onion, cook for ten minutes, stirring often.

Take the cooled garlic and grind it, then mixing it together with the cooked onion. Add the herbs and broth. Heat on medium heat until the soup begins to boil. Lower the heat and mix in bread, and cook for five minutes until the bread softens. Remove the herbs, place in a blender and blend until smooth. Add back to the soup. Add the sour cream, and salt and pepper to taste.

Turkey Chili

2 tablespoons olive oil
1 pound ground turkey
2 cups onions, chopped
1 cup red pepper, chopped
1 cup green pepper, chopped
2 cups celery, chopped
2 cloves garlic, chopped
2 tablespoons ground cumin
1 tablespoon chili powder
1 tablespoon paprika
1 teaspoon salt
Black pepper to taste
1 (15-ounce) can diced tomatoes
2 (15-ounce) cans red kidney beans
Cilantro, to taste (optional)
Scallions, to taste (optional)

Place the olive oil in a skillet. Add the turkey and onions. Cook until brown, about ten minutes. Add the remaining ingredients except cilantro and scallions. Simmer for thirty minutes. When finished, top with cilantro or scallions. Serve.

Turkey Stir-Fry

1 tablespoon vegetable oil
1 medium apple, chopped
1 small onion, chopped
1 clove garlic, minced
1/2 cup green pepper, diced
2 stalks celery, sliced thin
1 tablespoon butter
1 tablespoon whole-wheat flour
1 cup low-sodium chicken stock
1/4 teaspoon curry powder
1/2 teaspoon lime juice
1/4 teaspoon fresh ginger root, minced
2 cups cooked turkey breast, diced
1/2 teaspoon salt

Heat oil in large skillet on medium heat. Add the apple, onion, and garlic and cook until tender. Stir frequently. Add pepper and celery and stir-fry two minutes. Set aside.

In another large skillet, melt the butter and add the flour. Stir until golden brown. Then add chicken stock, curry, lime juice, and ginger. Heat through. Add previous mixture and turkey to the pan. Simmer for five minutes or until thoroughly heated through. Add salt to taste. Serve. Makes four servings.

Yeast Be Gone Soup

1 large yellow onion, peeled and sliced
4 stalks of celery, sliced
5 ounces of kale, or 4 to 5 cups
12 garlic cloves, sliced
Sea salt to taste
Water to cover vegetables in large pot

4 chicken breasts
Olive oil
Salt and pepper to taste

This recipe is great for a yeast infection or overgrowth of Candida. It is also great for killing cancer. Add the first six ingredients to a large stock pot. Add water. Cover and simmer until vegetables are tender, at least twenty minutes.

Place chicken breasts on cookie sheet and coat with olive oil. Salt and pepper to taste. Bake chicken at 350 degrees. Bake fresh chicken for twenty minutes or bake frozen chicken for forty minutes or until center of thickest piece is no longer pink. Once the chicken is cooked, remove from the oven and cut into small pieces and add to the vegetable mixture. Stir and serve.

Miscellaneous

Ant Zapper (Do Not Eat!)

1 empty water bottle
5 tablespoons aluminum-free baking soda
5 tablespoons powdered sugar
3 tablespoons water

Take the empty water bottle and cut it down to two inches tall, starting from the bottom. Mix the baking soda with the powdered sugar. You must use powdered sugar so it can mix well with the baking soda. You can mix it dry or add the water and stir well. Place small drops of the mixture on flat pieces of cardboard. Place the baited cardboard in the paths of the ants. They will take this back to the nest and share it with the queen and others to eat, killing off more ants. The acid in their stomachs reacts with the mixture, causing gas for the ants, which they can't expel.

Apricot-Banana Bread

2 medium bananas, mashed
4 whole dried apricots, chopped (8 halves)
1-1/2 cups whole-wheat flour
2 teaspoons baking powder
1/2 teaspoon salt
Dash nutmeg
1/3 cup vegetable oil
1/3 cup honey
1 egg

Combine the fruit in a small bowl. In second bowl, mix the flour, baking powder, salt, and nutmeg. Stir. Add the oil, honey, and egg. Beat well. Combine the two mixtures and stir well.

Grease the bottom and sides of a loaf pan (9-by-5-by-3-inches). Pour the batter in loaf pan to one-third full. Bake at 350 degrees for 35 minutes or until a toothpick inserted in the middle comes out clean. Serves ten.

Basic Simple Salad Dressing

1/3 cup olive oil
1/3 cup water
1/3 cup wine vinegar
2 cloves garlic, crushed
1/4 teaspoon salt
1 teaspoon dried tarragon
Fresh ground black pepper
1 teaspoon Dijon mustard (optional)
Dash of cayenne pepper (optional)

Place all ingredients in a jar with a lid. Shake ingredients and let stand for several hours. Shake before using. Store in refrigerator. If it turns solid, let sit at room temperature to liquefy or run jar under lukewarm water to warm contents slightly.

Basil Cell Carcinoma Killer

Aluminum-free baking soda
Raw organic coconut oil (Artisana brand recommended)
Antibiotic ointment

Mix one part baking soda with one part coconut oil. Add a half-inch line of antibiotic ointment to the mixture. Stir well in a small dish or jar. Apply the mixture to the affected area. Do not rub it in. Apply three applications a day for one week. Leave it on for thirty minutes if possible. For consecutive weeks of one to three applications a day, clean the area of dead skin before applying fresh ointment.

Cancer Buster

2 to 3 large ginger roots, finely ground
1-1/2 cups honey (from a reliable source so as not to have sugar in it)

Mix the ingredients together and store in a glass jar. Take a tablespoon three to four times a day. Use only a wooden or plastic spoon. You should experience good results in as little as four days. Reportedly, this should work on most cancers, especially ovarian and prostate. Early detection is key.

Cancer Kicker 2
(Alkaline Remedy)

2 teaspoons aluminum-free baking soda
1 teaspoon molasses
1 cup water

This recipe works well for prostate cancer, according to the My Dance With Cancer pH Kills Cancer website. Combine all ingredients, warm slightly, and stir. Drink this mix up to three times per day. Baking soda can raise your blood pressure, so if you suffer from high blood pressure, please check with your doctor before beginning this regimen. You should eliminate sugar in your diet. Read labels for sugar content. Cancer feeds off of sugar.

Cancer Kicker 3
(Alternative Alkaline Remedy)

3 teaspoons organic maple syrup
1 teaspoon aluminum-free baking soda (Red Mill brand recommended)

Combine ingredients in a small saucepan and stir over low heat (not over 120 degrees) for five to ten minutes. Take three teaspoons per day for one to two months. If it tastes bad, you burned it. Check your blood pressure regularly, as baking soda will raise it. Check with your doctor if you have high blood pressure.

Cinnamon Cancer Crusher

1 teaspoon Ceylon cinnamon
1 tablespoon honey

Mix together to make a paste. Consume this with bread, if desired. Consume three times a day for one month. Research in Japan and Australia revealed this mixture was helpful in advanced stomach and bone cancers. See Chapter 5 for cold prevention. This mixture is good for cancer, heart disease, arthritis, bladder infections, cholesterol, colds, upset stomach, gas, immune system, indigestion, influenza, longevity, sore throat, skin infections, weight loss, fatigue, bad breath, and hearing loss. To treat pimples, mix three tablespoons of honey with one teaspoon of cinnamon and apply to pimple. See Overall Good Health in Chapter 7 for more information.

Coleslaw and Dressing

3 tablespoons herbal vinegar of your choice
3 tablespoons virgin olive or coconut oil
2 to 3 tablespoons garlic honey
1/4 teaspoon mustard seed
1/4 teaspoon celery seed
1/4 teaspoon pepper
4 cups cabbage, shredded
1 cup carrots, shredded
1/2 cup celery, sliced

Mix the first six ingredients together in a small bowl. Place the cabbage, carrots, and celery in a large bowl and mix together. Pour the first mixture over the vegetable mixture and stir. Chill for 2 hours. Toss and serve.

Cricket Killer (Do Not Eat!)

2 small solid lids
Water
Cornmeal
Borax (optional)

Place one lid on the ground with water in it. Place the other lid about six inches away and put the cornmeal in it. The crickets will eat the cornmeal, get thirsty, go over to the water and have a drink. In a little bit of time, the crickets will explode because they cannot digest the two together. If this does not work, try adding a little bit of borax to the cornmeal.

Diabetes Defeat

1/2 teaspoon turmeric powder
1 teaspoon pure honey (no added glucose, starch, cane sugar, malt)
9 neem leaves (optional)

Mix together and serve daily. This recipe should help in the relief of diabetic symptoms. Sugar levels should be monitored before and after the consumption of honey if you are a diabetic.

Also, another remedy for diabetes relief is to take one tablespoon of the juice of the neem leaf daily first thing in the morning before eating anything. Reportedly, diabetes can be kept under control by consuming nine neem leaves daily.

Deodorant Recipe (Do Not Eat!)

6 to 8 tablespoons coconut oil (solid form)
1/4 cup aluminum-free baking soda
1/4 cup organic cornstarch or arrowroot powder

Mix ingredients together. Use empty deodorant container and fill it with deodorant or fill small jar with deodorant. Apply with container or fingers. Makes one cup.

Do-It-Yourself Deodorant Recipe (Do Not Eat!)

1 part aluminum-free baking soda
6 parts organic cornstarch or arrowroot powder
Shea butter (enough to make a paste)
A few drops of your favorite essential oil (such as
    rosemary or women's deodorant essential oil)

Mix together and store in a small, sealed jar. Apply with your fingertips daily
or as often as needed.

Donna's Fresh Ginger and Turmeric Relish

2 tablespoons fresh ginger, peeled and cut into thin rounds
2 tablespoons fresh turmeric, peeled and cut into thin rounds
2 tablespoons fresh white turmeric, peeled and
    cut into thin rounds (optional)
1 tablespoon chopped green chile
1/4 cup lime juice
1 teaspoon salt

Place all ingredients in a small bowl and mix well. Let the ingredients marinate
for two hours then serve. Store in an airtight container or a glass jar for up to
one week in the refrigerator.

Frozen Lemons

3 to 5 organic lemons with peel, washed

Place lemons in the freezer, peel and all. Once the citrus fruit is frozen, grate
and shred the whole lemon. Sprinkle on top of your meal. Goes great with
whiskey, wine, vegetable salad, soup, noodles, pastries, sorbets, spaghetti sauce,
rice, sushi, and fish dishes. The frozen lemon adds great flavor to your food.
The lemon peels add five to ten times more vitamins than the juice. Citrus
fruit helps to eliminate toxic elements in your body. Reportedly, lemon or
citrus fruits are fantastic at killing cancer cells, especially in the colon, breast,
prostate, lung, and pancreas.

Ginger Protocol

6 teaspoons of fresh ginger, grated
1 tablespoon raw honey (from a trusted producer with no added sugar)

Mix ginger and honey together. Consume six teaspoons of ginger every day for three days. Every couple of weeks repeat as needed or use three times a day for a stronger amount. This is great for shrinking tumors and fighting ovarian cancer and prostate cancer. Whole ginger extract has been known to shrink prostate tumors by 56 percent. Ginger has no toxicity in high doses. To order in bulk, go to the Starwest Botanicals website.

An alternative treatment is to take a few large ginger roots and grind them up. Then mix them with 1.1 pounds of honey from a trusted producer so there is no added sugar. Store in a glass jar and only use a wooden or plastic spoon to stir. Consume a tablespoon four times a day. One patient had success on her endocrine cancer with this protocol.

Honey and Ginger Treatment

1 (16-ounce) jar unpasteurized honey
1 (0.8-ounce) container ginger
1 (0.95-ounce) container turmeric

Honey is great at killing microbes inside cancer cells. On day one, take one teaspoon of honey with one teaspoon of turmeric. On day two, take one teaspoon of honey with one teaspoon of ginger. Continue alternating days with the turmeric and ginger.

Joint Inflammation Reduction

2 tablespoons cayenne pepper
1/2 cup coconut oil

Mix the ingredients together. Apply directly on the inflamed joint. Let it sit on the joint for at least twenty minutes. Repeat as often as needed.

Judy's Refrigerator Jam

1-1/3 cups strawberries
2/3 cup rhubarb
2 tablespoons raw honey (or to taste)
2 tablespoons chia seeds

Blend all ingredients together and place in the refrigerator overnight. The chia seeds will thicken into a gel-like substance. Add additional diced fruit for a thicker jam. Makes two cups.

Mice Exterminator (Do Not Eat!)

1 shallow lid
1 can sugary pop or soda

Place the drink in the lid. Set it along the edge of the wall where the rodents were last seen. Replace the liquid daily with fresh, bubbly, sugary pop. The mice cannot burp, and the carbonation kills them. DO NOT USE pop with artificial sweeteners. It is toxic to house pets.

Roach Exterminator (Do Not Eat!)

Boric acid (Ask your pharmacist where you can get this)
Flour or cornmeal

Mix half-and-half boric acid and flour. Place this powder in several lids and put the lids in the back of your kitchen sink cabinet, bathroom cabinets, and behind the refrigerator. Keep out of the reach of children and pets.

The Weed Exterminator (Do Not Eat!)

1 gallon vinegar
2 cups Epsom salt
1/4 cup liquid soap (like Dr. Bonner's)

Mix the ingredients in the morning and apply to weeds after the dew has disappeared. Check back in the evening, and the weeds should be expired. Be careful to spray this only on the plants you want to kill. You'll never buy toxic weed killers again.

Tom's Toothpaste

6 tablespoons aluminum-free baking soda
1 tablespoon 3 percent food-grade hydrogen peroxide
1 tablespoon melted coconut oil
Stevia
Spearmint oil for minty flavoring

Coconut oil is a great bacteria killer, which helps to avoid gum disease. Combine all of the ingredients together and store in a glass container.

Turmeric Topper

1 teaspoon turmeric powder
1 teaspoon olive oil
Generous pinch of fresh ground black pepper

Mix the ingredients together and add to vegetables, soups, and salad dressings. Use a tablespoon of fresh turmeric powder if you already have cancer.

Sides

Steamed asparagus
Steamed broccoli
Steamed cauliflower
Steamed cabbage
Green beans

Cheesy Cauliflower Patties

1 head cauliflower
1/2 cup cheddar cheese, grated
2 large eggs
1/2 cup Panko bread crumbs
1/2 teaspoon cayenne pepper, to taste
Salt to taste
Olive oil

Clean and cut cauliflower into little pieces and boil in water until tender, approximately ten minutes. Drain. Mash. Stir in the rest of the ingredients except the olive oil.

Coat the skillet with olive oil. Heat to medium-high heat. Shape the mixture into three-inch patties and cook until golden brown, approximately three minutes per side. Keep each batch warm in the oven while cooking the rest.

Creamy Asparagus

16 ounces or 1 pound fresh asparagus
1/2 cup water
1 onion, chopped
1 can cream of mushroom soup
2 tablespoons butter
1 cup baby bella mushrooms, sliced
4 ounces cheddar cheese, shredded

Cook asparagus in water in saucepan until crisp-tender. In skillet, sauté onions and mushrooms until wilted. Add mushroom soup. Stir. Add cheese. Stir until melted. Remove from heat and pour over asparagus. Serve.

Chicken Apple Salad

1 serving precooked chicken breast, diced
1 apple, diced
1 cup celery, diced
1/4 cup water
1/2 teaspoon curry powder
Dash of garlic powder
Dash of onion powder
Dash of cayenne
Dash of cinnamon
Salt and pepper to taste
1 packet of Stevia, optional

Combine first three ingredients in a large bowl. In another pan, heat the water and add remaining ingredients. Stir. Pour spicy mixture over chicken, apple, and celery mixture. Chill at least one hour in the refrigerator before serving.

Fruit Salad

1 quart fresh strawberries, stemmed and halved
1 (20-ounce) can pineapple chunks, drained
4 firm bananas, sliced
1 (11-ounce) can mandarin orange slices, drained

Gently mix all ingredients together. Chill for one hour. Serve.

Green Beans and Garlic

16 ounces green beans, ends trimmed
1 cup water
2 tablespoons butter
1 cup baby bella mushrooms, sliced
1/2 teaspoon garlic, chopped
1/2 teaspoon salt
1/4 teaspoon pepper
1 teaspoon dried oregano
1/3 cup shredded Parmesan cheese
1 pound turkey bacon, cooked and crumbled (optional) (Beeler's brand)

Pour water in pan. Add beans and cover saucepan. Cook until crisp-tender. Drain. Add butter to skillet. Sauté mushrooms and garlic in butter. Add beans and sauté until heated through. Add oregano, salt, and pepper to taste. Before serving, top with crumbled bacon and shredded cheese.

Jalapeno Poppers
(Very alkaline recipe)

1 cup pine nuts
6 medium pitted dates
2 tablespoons apple cider vinegar
1/2 clove garlic
1 large avocado
1 teaspoon Celtic sea salt
1 tablespoon lemon juice
16 Jalapeno peppers

Blend the pine nuts, dates, vinegar, and garlic in a food processor until smooth. Add the soft insides of the avocado to the mix. Blend. Add sea salt and lemon juice to the mix and blend lightly.

Wear disposable gloves when cutting pepper tops off and discarding the seeds. Slit the sides of the peppers for stuffing if needed. Fill the peppers with stuffing mix. Place the peppers on a baking sheet. Bake the peppers for five hours at 105 degrees to dehydrate them. Serve warm. Great healthy finger food. Enjoy! This recipe includes many alkaline ingredients. This is great for getting your body to fight off bacteria and viruses.

Spinach Salad

8 ounces fresh spinach leaves, washed
1/2 cup chopped walnuts
1 cup fresh strawberries, sliced
1 small can mandarin oranges, drained

Recipe continues with Oil and Vinegar Dressing.

Oil and Vinegar Dressing

3/4 cup olive oil
1/4 cup cider vinegar

Mix oil and vinegar together in small container. Mix remaining ingredients together and pour dressing over spinach salad.

Spinach Side Salad

2 cups spinach, washed
1/2 cup cucumbers, sliced
1 small tomato, sliced
2 hard-cooked eggs, sliced
4 ounces cheddar cheese, shredded
Ranch dressing or oil/vinegar dressing

Place ingredients on serving plate, in order listed. Top with ranch dressing or oil and vinegar dressing. See recipe for oil and vinegar dressing above. Serves two.

Veggie Medley

1-1/2 cups raw broccoli, cut up
1-1/2 cups raw zucchini, cut up
1/2 cup raw sweet red pepper, cut up
1/4 cup raw onion, cut up
2 tablespoons butter
2 tablespoons chicken broth

Combine ingredients in a microwave-safe, quart-sized dish. Cover and microwave for four minutes until tender-crisp. Let stand for a few minutes. Serve.

Healthy Snack Attacks

Eat organic berries. Anything that has the words berries or berry in its name is a great snack for cancer patients. Seeds contain vitamin B17, which is great at killing cancer cells. Berries have seeds, so stock up on berries. Citrus fruits are known to kill cancer cells as well. Also, raw nuts such as organic walnuts, almonds, sunflower seeds, hemp seeds, etc., are great for adding healthy fats to your diet to protect your joints and skin.

Smoothies

If the cold bothers you due to chemotherapy treatments, let the ingredients warm up to room temperature and then blend. If the recipe calls for ice, substitute room temperature water. The main point is to get the nutrition in your body so it can help boost your immune system. Add a bitter apricot kernel to any smoothie. It's great for killing cancer.

Berry Fruit Smoothie
(Alkaline Drink)

2 medium to large ripe bananas
2 cups frozen mixed berries (blackberry, blueberry, raspberry, or
    strawberry)
1 to 2 cups kale (remove the spine - any variety will work)
2 to 3 tablespoons raw pumpkin seeds
1/2 to 1 cup of purified water

Place all ingredients in a medium-speed blender and blend until smooth.

Berry Burst

This detoxification drink is bursting with antioxidants. The fat and protein keeps you feeling full and sustains your energy.

2 cups unsweetened almond milk
1-1/2 bananas, frozen and broken into chunks
2 cups baby spinach
1 cup blueberries, frozen
2 tablespoons almond butter
1 tablespoon chia seeds
1 cup ice

Pour the almond milk in the blender first. Add remaining ingredients and blend until creamy. Pour into a glass. Serve.

Berry Smoothie

2 cups organic coconut milk, unsweetened
1 cup mixed berries
1 frozen banana
1 scoop vanilla protein powder (rBGH free) (grass-fed if possible)

Blend ingredients together until smooth. Pour into a glass and enjoy!

Fall Smoothie

4 apples, sliced
Water
1/2 lemon, juiced
4 to 5 kale leaves

Blend apples with water. Add the lemon juice and kale leaves and blend some more. Serve.

Chocolate Blast
(Great for breakfast or anytime! This recipe featured on the front cover.)

1 cup organic unsweetened vanilla almond, coconut, or cashew milk
1 tablespoon organic coconut oil or flaxseed oil
3 teaspoons unsweetened cocoa powder
2 tablespoons vanilla protein powder (grass fed is best) or 1 scoop
1-1/2 tablespoons avocado flesh (optional)
2 to 3 dashes cinnamon (optional) (helps regulate blood sugar)
2 tablespoons organic almond butter (freshly ground has no sugar)
1 small handful of raw spinach (optional)
1 small organic banana, sliced and frozen, or 25 slices frozen banana
2 dates, pitted, chopped (optional)
Whipped cream spray topping (optional)

A hand blender works well for this recipe. Note: Cashew milk seems to make the recipe creamier. Add milk of choice to the blender or bowl. Add remaining ingredients except banana and dates. Blend well. Add frozen banana in chunks and blend until creamy. Add dates and blend. Enjoy with whipped topping.

Lean, Mean, Green Smoothie Machine

1 large handful kale, chopped
1 celery stalk
1 large handful spinach
1/2 lemon, peeled
1-inch fresh ginger, peeled
1 teaspoon apple cider vinegar
4 pineapple chunks (approximately 1-1/2 inches square)
1 cup water (more if needed)

In a blender, blend all ingredients until smooth. Pour into a glass and enjoy!

Protein Smoothie

1/2 cup unsweetened cashew or almond milk
1/2 cup fresh or frozen blueberries
2 scoops chocolate protein powder
1/2 medium-sized frozen banana

You can slice and freeze the other half of the banana and save it for the next time. Blend ingredients. If too thick, add more milk.

Skin Booster Smoothie

1/2 lemon
1 handful cilantro
1 cup purslane (or kale or spinach)
1 cucumber
1/2 mango, sliced

Place lemon, cilantro, purslane, and cucumber in blender or juicer. Blend. Add slices of mango piece by piece until thoroughly blended. This is a great detoxification drink.

Spring Smoothie

1 handful wild dandelion greens (best in the spring when tender)
1 small handful mint leaves
3 cups honeydew melon

Make sure the greens have not been sprayed. Blend together and serve.

Strawberry Nana Smoothie

1 cup strawberries, stemmed and washed
1 frozen banana, in pieces
1/2 to 1 cup orange juice

Blend until smooth. If too thick, add more juice and blend again. Serve.

Summer Smoothie

1 cup fresh orange juice
1 ripe frozen banana
1 cup frozen mangoes
1 large handful kale

If you prefer a thicker smoothie, add more banana and mangoes. Delicious!

The Pick-Me-Up

2-1/2 cups unsweetened almond coconut milk
2 cups mango chunks
2 bananas, frozen and broken into chunks
2 cups spinach
2 tablespoons shredded coconut
1 cup ice
2 tablespoons pea protein powder

Pea protein powder is a high-quality protein powder that works great for people with allergies to animal protein. This is a great detoxification drink.

Pour almond coconut milk in blender. Add remaining ingredients. Blend until smooth.

Winter Smoothie

1 cup organic frozen berries (preferably red)
Water (just enough to be able to blend everything together, about 1 cup)
2 cups fresh spinach (green)
1/4-inch fresh ginger, peeled

Blend the berries with water first. Add the spinach and ginger, blend. Savor.

Chapter 10
Powerhouse Cancer Fighting Foods

The foods listed in this chapter are great to add to your diet in moderation. These foods boost your immune system. Always use organic whenever possible. If you are currently under the care of a physician for cancer or otherwise, please check with your doctor for medical interactions with the foods listed in this chapter. If you cannot find any of these products in your area, check Chapter 11.

Acai Berry: Due to its antioxidant effects, there may be certain interactions with some chemotherapy drugs. Check with your doctor first. Laboratory studies show that flavonoids in acai fruit have antioxidant properties.

AHCC (Active Hexose Correlated Compound)/Mushrooms: This is a proprietary medicinal mushroom extract intended to strengthen the immune system. The formula is a trade secret of the Japanese manufacturer. However, we do know that several species of Basidiomycete mushrooms, including shiitake mushrooms, have been shown to exhibit anticancer effects. A medical doctor suggested these mushrooms for their anticancer effects: Turkey Tail (use liquid or encapsulated extracts), Maitake (aka hen of the woods), Reishi (teabags, capsules, and liquid extracts), and/or Agaricus blazei (dried or extracts).

Other medicinal mushrooms besides shiitake are maitake, cordyceps, reishi coriolus, and phellinus linteus. They have found that these mushrooms have extended survival times and work best on breast, lung, and prostate cancers. Able to shrink tumors by up to 70 percent, some extracts make cancers disappear altogether. They stimulate the immune system, reduce blood supply to tumors, and reduce cancer treatment side effects such as nausea and hair loss. An extract of astragalus and vitamin D are great additions to your diet and help to beat cancer. Studies have shown that long-term consumption of reishi mushrooms prevents the spread of cancerous tumors and increases the antioxidants in blood plasma.

Many people have had good luck in helping their cancer with a product called "Noxylane." It is a derivative of shiitake mushroom enzymes and Heated Algal Ingredient (HAI™).

Alliums: (Onions, garlic, shallots, chives, and leeks) These vegetables contain a sulfur compound that protects against carcinogens and makes cancer cells die. These vegetables help defeat colon, breast, lung, and prostate cancer cells.

Garlic also helps lower your risk for kidney, stomach, brain, lung, and prostate cancers. Garlic kills brain cancer cells without side effects. The active compounds in garlic are released when you crush the clove. The crushed garlic can be absorbed easily when added to oil. It also can be eaten raw, added to salads, or layered in sandwiches. Garlic's active ingredients, selenium, tryptophan, and sulfur-based agents, attack cancer cells. The key is to let the crushed garlic sit for fifteen minutes before use to release the anticancer compounds.

Aloe Vera: Research shows strong immunomodulatory and antitumor properties for aloe vera. It also is known to boost immunity and destroy cancer tumors. Aloe is edible, but the green outer skin may be unpalatable to some. Many people consume it poached or steamed before adding it to a salad, juice, soup, or stir-fry.

Apricot Kernels: Apricot kernels provide amygdalin, otherwise known as vitamin B17. You won't find this vitamin in the store. Everyone's nutritional needs are different, and it is not recommended to consume more than three kernels per hour with a maximum of ten per day. Follow recommended dosages on the package.

If you are taking laetrile tablets and kernels, wait two hours between taking them. The kernels (found inside the hard seed) attack cancer cells and aid in the prevention of cancer cells in our bodies and may also lower blood pressure. Start with a small dose if you have low blood pressure. Dr. Ernst T. Krebs Jr., a biochemist, first produced a concentrated amygdalin (laetrile) in the 1950s. He claimed that if you consumed ten to twelve apricot kernels daily, you would be cancer free unless you were exposed to high concentrations of nuclear radiation. Great excitement in the 1950s showed that laetrile (concentrated nitriloside compound from the apricot kernel) worked at killing cancer, but if it could not be made into a drug, the cancer industry would collapse and no money could be made. Laetrile stopped the spread of cancer in mice and the growth of tumors. It also showed that it acted as a great cancer preventer.

Amygdalin / Vitamin B17:   This is recommended as an add-on supplement in the fight against cancer. The Anti-Cancer Info website from the United Kingdom offers an interesting article called, "The Role of Vitamin B17 in the Fight Against Cancer." Vitamin B17 is found in the seeds or kernels of the following: apricot seeds (the kernel), nectarine seeds, pear seeds, prune seeds, squash seeds, apple pips (seeds), peach kernels, plum kernels, fava beans, garbanzo beans, cashew (low), grape seeds, nectarine kernels, cherry kernels, boysenberry, choke cherry, elderberry, raspberry, mulberry, millet, flax, wild crabapple, beans, pulses, bitter almonds, alfalfa leaves, eucalyptus leaves, bamboo sprouts, Swedish lingonberries, cranberry, macadamia nuts, and grains (if not highly hybridized). Sprouts rich in vitamin B17 are bamboo, millet, and alfalfa sprouts. I would warn not to overdose on these seeds. Start by eating no more seeds than what can be found in one fruit. If you purchase these seeds or kernels, only consume what the package recommends. Talk to your doctor about amygdalin injectable options. Amygdalin has been found to inhibit tumor effects in animals. Although not proven, it is thought that normal cells convert cyanide to benign thiocynate via rhodanese (a mitochondrial enzyme that detoxifies cyanide) in humans. It has been reported that vitamin B17 works well for benign tumors, cysts, and warts.

Avocados: Avocados posses a lipid called avocatin B, which targets leukemia stem cells, according to a Canadian professor Paul Spagnuolo. The Aztecs referred to avocados as the "fertility fruit." Just saying, you've been warned! Keep avocados away from your dog as the seed can get stuck in the esophagus, stomach, or intestinal tract. Also, keep avocados away from horses, cattle, and birds. It can be toxic to these animals.

Beetroot: Beetroot and other purple-colored fruits and vegetables contain anthocyanins and some resveratrol that kills cancer cells. It is great in fighting blood and brain cancers. Beetroot extracts increase the nitric oxide levels in your blood stream, which relaxes the blood vessels, lowering your blood pressure and indirectly helping with erectile dysfunction.

Berries: Berries with seeds in or on them—such as blueberries, huckleberries, boysenberries, elderberries, gooseberries, loganberries, mulberries, strawberries, raspberries, blackberries, cranberries, cherries, etc.—are the key. Eat the seeds because they contain vitamin B17, aka laetrile, which helps stop the replication of cancer cells and build immunity. If you already have cancer, you should consider vitamin B17 in conjunction with other treatment methods. Anthocyanidins and proanthocyanidins promote cancer cell death. Frozen berries are just as strong as fresh.

Ripe organic strawberries dipped in dark chocolate act as a double weapon in killing cancer cells. Stick to the dark chocolate that has very little sugar in it for best results. Remember, cancer feeds off of sugar.

Elderberries are potent antiviral fruits. Native Americans used these berries for boosting their immune system. Keep in mind that in raw form, elderberries are poisonous and need to be cooked and properly prepared before consumption. Elderberry juice extract is excellent for colds and flu prevention.

A colorectal cancer study at the University of Colorado Cancer Center showed that black raspberries decreased new tumors by 45 percent and decreased existing tumors by 60 percent. Additional research showed that berries, grapes, and apples reduced the risk of colon cancer.

Brazil Nuts: Six nuts will give you five hundred and forty-four micrograms of selenium. Recommended daily dosage is fifty-five micrograms, or two nuts.

Do not consume more than six nuts per day, but if you are eating them daily, eat only one or two nuts per day. Consuming too many nuts in one sitting can lead to selenium toxicity. Selenium is very potent at killing cancer cells.

Carrots: Cooked carrots are packed with lots of healthy nutrients when it comes to fighting cancer as well as apricots, peppers, and pumpkins. They are helpful in slowing the growth of cancer and protect cell membranes from toxins. Carrots are helpful in fighting mouth, esophagus, stomach, and cervical cancers. Note: Use caution in eating too many carrots if you already have certain cancers because they may spike your insulin, and cancer feeds off of sugar.

Chia Seeds: One teaspoon of chia seed contains two-and-a-half more protein than kidney beans, three times more antioxidants than blueberries, three times more iron than spinach, six times more calcium than milk, seven times more vitamin C than oranges, eight times more omega-3 than salmon, ten times more fiber than rice, and fifteen times more magnesium than broccoli. The seeds also are gluten-free, help reduce joint pain, aid in weight loss, provide an energy boost, and guard against diabetes and heart disease. See Judy's Refrigerator Jam in Chapter 10.

Citrus Fruits: Lemons, lime, oranges, grapefruit, tangerines, and pineapple contain anti-inflammatory compounds called flavonoids that prompt the liver to detoxify carcinogens. The skins of tangerines contain tangeritin and nobiletin, which help to kill brain cancer cells. Simply grate the organic skins into salads, breakfast cereals, hot tea, or a salsa to season grilled fish. Eat at least two to three citrus fruits a day if you have cancer. When my mother did this, a biopsy showed dead cancer cells. Mix up the fruits to gain the advantage of what all the fruits and berries have to offer.

Crucifers: (Broccoli, cauliflower, Brussels sprouts, kale, and cabbage family) Crucifers protect against estrogen, one of the many hormones that signal cancer cells to grow. The cruciferous vegetables help eliminate toxins. Michigan State University research found that those who ate raw or lightly cooked cabbage and sauerkraut three times a week or more were 72 percent less likely to get breast cancer. Five weekly half-cup servings is a reasonable goal. Crucifers are great at fighting estrogen-driven cancers like breast, uterine lining, lung, colon, liver, cervix, prostate, brain, stomach, and colorectal.

Dark Chocolate: The dark chocolates with 70 percent or more cocoa provide a number of antioxidants, proanthocyanidins, and polyphenols. One square (about one-fifth of a bar) of dark chocolate contains double the amount of antioxidants as a red glass of wine and almost the equivalent of a cup of steeped green tea. These molecules slow the growth of cancer cells and limit the blood vessels that feed them. The dairy in milk chocolate cancels the protection of the polyphenol compounds.

Dark Leafy Greens and Vital Vegetables: According to the American Institute for Cancer Research, dark green leafy vegetables are good at fighting cancer. These vegetables include spinach, kale, romaine lettuce, leaf lettuce, mustard greens, collard greens, chicory, and Swiss chard. Laboratory research has concluded that the carotenoids can inhibit the growth of certain types of breast cancer cells, skin cancer cells, lung cancer, and stomach cancer. Spinach removes free radicals from your body before they damage it. It is considered the most nutrient-dense green vegetable. Raw or slightly cooked spinach is found to protect against mouth, esophagus, ovarian, endometrial, lung, colorectal, and stomach cancer.

Folate helps your body produce new cells and repair DNA.

Vegetables such as Brussels sprouts, bok choy, Chinese cabbage, broccoli, and cauliflower have sulforaphane and indole-3-carbinols that are anticancer molecules. These molecules kill off cancer cells and block tumor growth.

When preparing these vegetables, cover them and only steam them briefly or stir-fry quickly with a little olive oil. Avoid boiling the vegetables because it destroys the anticancer molecules.

Dry Beans: Dry beans are considered lentils, chickpeas, beans, soya, pinto beans, navy beans, dry peas, and others. They are sometimes referred to as pulses or grain legumes. Pulses contain isoflavones and phytoestrogens. Plant estrogens are forty to fifty times less potent than human estrogen. Dry beans provide fibers that help neutralize free radicals in the gut and blood stream. Eat beans about twice a week.

Egg Yolks: Egg yolks contain folic acid along with green leafy vegetables; avocados, beans, carrots, apricots, whole grains, and pumpkins—and is great at protecting your DNA during radiotherapy. Four hundred micrograms is the recommended serving. Refer to the food sources chart on the Florida Folic Acid Coalition website for food serving sizes.

Ginger: The American Association for Cancer Research showed that ginger helps with inflammation and nausea. When using ginger powder, cancer cells died, according to a study at the University of Michigan. This has been helpful for prostate and ovarian cancer. Whole ginger extract shrunk a prostate tumor by 56 percent. Check with your doctor before taking ginger if you are pregnant.

Goji Berries: Goji berries are a natural option in the fight against cancer. They work by cutting off the blood supply to the cancer cells. A 1994 study with seventy-nine cancer patients found they responded better to their cancer treatment when Goji berries were added to their diet. The cyperone, physalin, and selenium found in the berries helps to treat cervical cancer, breast cancer, leukemia, testicular cancer, lung cancer, liver cancer, colon, prostate, gastric, and uterine cancer.

These berries contain eighteen amino acids, eight essential acids, twenty-one trace minerals, and trace amounts of zinc, copper, iron, magnesium, selenium, manganese, and phosphorous, vitamins A, C, E, B1, B2 and B6, essential fatty acids like omega-3 and omega-6, and many anti-inflammatory, antifungal, and antibacterial agents.

The berries can be added to cereals, salads, soups, baked goods, trail mixes, and smoothies, and made into a tea. Their taste is tangy sweet and sour and make for a great substitute for raisins in recipes.

Grass-fed Beef: If you like to eat beef, grass-fed beef or grass-fed buffalo would be your best options. The Eskimos who consumed 100 percent meat in their diets (at certain times of the year) were reportedly cancer-free. Why? They ate a lot of caribou and other animals that ate grass. Vitamin B17 contains nitrolosides or laetrile, which occurs naturally in about eighteen hundred plants. Grass is one of those eighteen hundred plants that are high in cancer-fighting nitrolosides, which explains why grass-fed beef, buffalo, or caribou is a much better option for you.

Green Tea: The Mayo Clinic in Rochester, Minnesota, states that three to five cups a day can inhibit cancer cell growth.

Ground Flax Seeds: Ground flax seeds have been shown to reduce tumor growth in animals and have the potential for minimizing the risk of developing breast and prostate cancer in humans. These are great for adding to cereals, baked goods, and smoothies. If they are left whole, they pass through the body without much benefit.

Iodine: The lack of iodine has been implicated in many patients as the culprit in causing breast and ovarian cancer. Many food manufacturers and processors are turning to sea salt in their products instead of iodized salt, which puts more people at risk for iodine deficiency. If you don't have enough iodine in your diet, your body can't make enough thyroid hormone. A deficiency in your body leads to enlargement of the thyroid (or goiter), hypothyroidism, and to mental retardation in infants and children whose mothers were iodine deficient during pregnancy. Sources of dietary iodine include cheese, cow's milk, eggs, frozen yogurt, ice cream, iodine-containing multivitamins, iodized table salt, saltwater fish, seaweed, shellfish, soy milk, soy sauce, and yogurt.

Multi-strain Probiotic: It is recommended you take a daily probiotic. When people are going to travel out of the country, some doctors will prescribe a strong probiotic, which helps people combat any bacteria or viruses they will encounter. Without the right bacteria in your gut, your body won't reap the benefits of all the healthy foods you'll be eating. Remember to avoid salt and sugar (glucose) since cancer cells feed off of sugar. Healthy cells can use fat cells for energy.

Oil of Oregano: Oregano is known to be a powerhouse natural antibiotic and effective antiviral herb. It also boasts healing properties. Oregano contains eight times the natural antibiotics of apples and three times that of blueberries. This natural antioxidant protects your body against free radical damage and boosts your own body's immune system.

Oregano oil is very potent and is antiviral, antibacterial, antiseptic, anti-fungal, and anti-inflammatory. Hippocrates was a highly regarded, ancient Greek physician. One of the main tools he used for antibacterial use was oregano oil. Leaves of the oregano plant are great for the respiratory and digestive systems.

Oily Fish: Fish oil provides omega-3, vitamin A, and a little vitamin D. Vitamins A and D are important against the fight of cancer. Fish that provide rich oils are herring, mackerel, and salmon. Fish oils help in the fight against prostate, breast, and colon cancer.

Parsley: In a 2013 test, a compound found in parsley killed 86% of lung cancer cells in a laboratory Petri dish. The plant-derived flavonoid that kills cancer cells is called apigenin, and it can be found not only in parsley but celery and onions, too. Parsley also has been used to treat or break up kidney stones.

Peaches: According to research at Washington State University with Texas A & M, polyphenol chemicals in peaches kill metastatic cancer cells in breast cancer. When the peaches are ingested, it signals metastatic cancer cells to kill themselves. The researchers suggested that a high-dose peach extract would offer great advances in the treatment of cancer. It is suggested that the peaches with the most red in them offer the most benefits. Rich Lady was the type of peach used in the study. Other red peaches are Crest Haven, Red Haven, Elberta, and Blushing Star.

Pomegranate Seeds: Rich in antioxidants, vitamin C, and potassium, pome-granate seeds and juice pump up the level of oxygen in your blood, prevent hardening of the artery walls with excess fat, and help reduce the risk of cancer and heart disease. It has a higher antioxidant activity than green tea or red wine.

Pumpkin Seeds: Five tablespoons daily will provide twenty milligrams of vitamin E and inhibit cancer cell growth. Recommended dosage is three hundred to six hundred milligrams but is hard to achieve without supplements. Good sources are green vegetables, soya, and almonds. Pumpkin seeds are alkaline-forming and can reduce levels of LDL cholesterol. Anti-inflammatory, they reduce arthritis and kidney stone formation. The seeds are an excellent remedy for prostate health and good sleep. They are filled with minerals and zinc.

Red and Yellow Peppers: Red and yellow peppers are ranked as a top source of vitamin C in the United Kingdom. Vitamin C boosts your immune system and helps to neutralize toxins. It is recommended to eat 10 grams or two teaspoons daily. A large red pepper is 250 milligrams of vitamin C.

Ripe Bananas: Japanese scientific research shows that a ripe banana with dark spots enhances your immunity and possesses an anticancer quality. The ripe banana is eight times more effective at enhancing the white blood cells. Ripe bananas are rich in alkaline minerals such as potassium, magnesium, calcium, selenium, vitamin C, and vitamin E. Ripe bananas can easily be sliced, frozen, and used for smoothies.

Spices and Herbs: Spices and herbs have anticancer benefits. Both fresh and dried are great at suppressing cancer growth. Spruce up your meals with basil, rosemary, parsley, mint, cinnamon, cardamom, ginger, and turmeric with black pepper and olive oil. Also, garlic and lemon balm have strong antiviral and antibacterial properties. Lemon balm is effective in fighting the flu, colds, chicken pox, or shingles. Lemon balm oil is prescribed overseas for sufferers of herpes or cold sores. Lemon balm comes in the form of a cream, tincture, and tea. Check with your doctor if you are pregnant or considering using lemon balm while on medication.

Top Six Alkaline Foods for Daily Use: Root vegetables (radishes, beets, carrots, turnips, horseradish, and rutabagas), cruciferous vegetables (broccoli, cabbage, cauliflower, Brussels sprouts, etc.), leafy greens (kale, Swiss chard, turnip greens, and spinach), garlic, cayenne peppers, and lemons. Note: Skip carrots if you already have cancer. They may increase your insulin, and cancer feeds off of sugar.

Turmeric Spice: Turmeric cleanses infections, reduces inflammation and helps with joint pain. It also prevents dementia and blocks the advancement of cancer. Some research shows it is more effective when it's mixed with black pepper and dissolved in olive oil. If purchased directly from a spice shop, the fresh spice is stronger. In South Asia, turmeric is added to warm milk to relieve digestive problems, cold symptoms, a cough, or a sore throat. When added to pharmaceutical treatments, turmeric is a complementary treatment for cancer, cirrhosis, chronic kidney disease, chronic obstructive lung disease, diabetes, and Alzheimer's. Fresh turmeric works better and enhances chemotherapy. See Chapter 10 for turmeric recipes.

Prepared yellow mustard contains turmeric spice in it. My grandmother lived to 105 cancer-free, and she always loved potato salad. The potato salad she ate contained a lot of yellow mustard. I can't say with 100 percent certainty, but it sure makes me wonder if the turmeric in mustard helped to protect her from cancer. She also worked hard and ate healthy, homegrown foods.

Sunflower Seeds: An excellent source of magnesium and vitamin E, sunflower seeds help to neutralize free radicals. In sufficient amounts, they enhance your immunity and reduce your risk of certain cancers. The salt-free seeds also lower your blood pressure, prevent migraine headaches, reduce heart attacks, and prevent strokes. They are high in vitamin E and zinc. Zinc and vitamin C work together to speed healing time. Sunflower seeds are great for prostate health. Seven tablespoons or more are recommended per day.

Tomatoes: The red color from tomatoes comes from a phytochemical called lycopene, a powerhouse antioxidant. Studies show that a lycopene-rich diet can reduce the risk of prostate cancer. It also prevents the growth of cancer cells in breast, lung, colon, cervix, and endometrial tissue. Processing or cooking the tomatoes activates the cancer-fighting compounds to protect your body. Other foods that contain lycopene are watermelon, pink grapefruit, and red bell peppers. Harvard research suggests seven to ten helpings per week, especially cooked. The red coloring contains lycopene, which reduces fat levels and is a strong antioxidant.

Whole Grains: Look for "100 percent whole organic wheat." If available, look for bread sprinkled with flax or sesame seeds. Diets high in fiber (vegetables and fruits included) have a lower risk of colorectal cancer.

Finale

Foods have cancer-fighting properties. Avoiding cancer and fighting cancer is like fighting a fire. You need many fire trucks or, in this case, many different foods and protocols to fight cancer. A healthy diet filled with colorful fruits and vegetables is the key to avoiding heart disease, diabetes, and diet-induced cancer. Foods such as broccoli, berries, citrus fruits, seeds, kernels, and garlic provide the biggest boosts to cancer prevention. Phytochemicals from cruciferous vegetables protect our cells from harmful compounds found in our food and in the environment.

Eating well doesn't have to be expensive. Check out your local farmer's market, organic grocery stores, or order from the suppliers listed in Chapter 11. Stock up on organic foods that are on sale, or buy them in bulk and save with quantity discounts. You can also plant a small garden in buckets with drain holes, large pots, raised garden beds, or community gardens. Plant a fruit tree or bush. Asparagus comes back year-after-year.

Plenty of fruits and vegetables, whole grains, and lean meat or fish will be a powerhouse in keeping you healthy and feeling well. Cut back on carbs and sugar. Also, throw in some exercise into your routine. Take a fifteen-minute walk.

I hope this book inspires you to feel empowered to take preventative measures now. If you ever receive or have received a cancer diagnosis, it will help you to be informed of the choices you have in the battle against cancer. You do have options. What are you waiting for? Go grab an orange!

If you found this book to be of value to you, please leave a review online. It will help others in the fight against cancer. Thank you!

Chapter 11
Organic Food and Seed Suppliers

Healthy cooking doesn't have to be complicated or hard. Make enough so you don't have to cook every night. Freeze some meals in advance for those nights you are short on time. Note: The country calling code for the United States and Canada is 1.

Specialty Foods

www.eatwild.com
The Eatwild Store
State-by-state pastured products

www.applegate.com
Natural and organic meats

www.organickitchen.com
Nationwide products

www.orgfood.com
Organic provisions
(Beans, flours, grains, seeds, nuts, dried fruits)

www.sunorganic.com
Sun Organic Farm products

**Small Package and
Grocery Organic Suppliers**

www.spicely.com
Spicely Organics
(Showroom location)
578 Market Street
San Francisco, CA 94104
(415) 982-7742

Oilerie Maple Grove
13551 Grove Drive
Maple Grove, MN 55311
(763) 657-0857

Whole Foods (Metcalf)
7401 West 91st Street
Overland Park, KS 66212
(913) 652-9633

Whole Foods (Overland Park)
6621 W. 119th Street
Overland Park, KS 66209
(913) 663-2951

Oilerie Fish Creek
4083 Main Street
P. O. Box 31
Fish Creek, WI 54212
(800) 310-2878

Andersons Market #39
P. O. Box 119
Maumee, OH 43537
(419) 891-2700

Anderson's Market #41
4701 Talmadge Road
Toledo, OH 43623
(419) 473-3232

Whole Foods (Sandy Springs)
5930 Roswell Road
Atlanta, GA 30328
(404) 236-0810

Whole Foods (Asheville)
70 Merrimon Avenue
Asheville, NC 28801
(828) 254-5440

Akins Natural Foods -
  Site 5 Elk River Trading
7807 East 51st
Tulsa, OK 74145
(918) 663-4137

Whole Foods
  (Franklin, TN-McEwen)
1566 West McEwen Drive
Franklin, TN 37067
(615) 550-5660

Whole Foods (Alpharetta)
1180 Upper Hembree Road
Roswell, GA 30076
(770) 667-8878

Whole Foods
  (Marietta, GA - Merchants Walk)
1131 Johnson Ferry Road
Marietta, GA 30068
(678) 996-9700

The Oilerie Hilton Head Island
1000 William Hilton Parkway
Hilton Head Island, 29928
(843) 681-2722

Whole Foods (Duluth)
5945 State Bridge Road
Duluth, GA 30097
(678) 514-2400

Whole Foods (Birmingham)
3100 Cahaba Village Plaza
Birmingham, AL 35243
(205) 912-8400

Whole Foods
  (Nashville-Greenhills)
4021 Hillsboro Pike
Nashville, TN 37215
(615) 440-5100

New Pioneer Food Co-op
22 S. Van Buren
Iowa City, IA 52240
(319) 338-9441

New Pioneer Food Co-op
1101 2nd Street
Coralville, IA 52241
(319) 358-5513

New Pioneer Food Co-op
3338 Center Point Road NE
Cedar Rapids, IA 52402
(319) 365-2632

Bulk Food Organic Suppliers

www.shoporganic.com
Email:
customerservice@shoporganic.com
shopOrganic
3450 S. Broadmont Drive
Suite 114
Tucson, AZ 85713

www.frontiercoop.com
Email:
customercare@frontiercoop.com
Frontier Natural Products Co-op
P. O. Box 299
3021 78th St.
Norway, IA 52318
Phone: (800) 669-3275

www.gardenspotdist.com
Garden Spot Distributors
191 Commerce Drive
New Holland, PA 17557
Phone: (717) 354-4936

www.sunfood.com
Sunfood Super Foods
1830 Gillespie Way, Suite 101
El Cajon, CA 92020
Phone: (619) 596-7979

www.albertsorganics.com
Albert's Organics
Albert's East Division
1155 Commerce Blvd.
Logan Township, NJ 08085
Phone: (800) 899-5944 x63136
Note: There are seven divisions across the United States. Call and ask for the division nearest to you or check the website.

www.naturalgrocers.com
Natural Grocers
400 N Stadium Blvd
Columbia, MO 65203

Note: There are grocers in fifteen states. Call and ask for the one located closest to you or check the website.

www.organicwholesaleclub.com
Organic Wholesale Club
3020 Issaquah Pine-Lake Road, 514
Sammamish, WA 98075
Phone: (425) 369-9209

Seed Suppliers

www.seedsavers.org
Email: Online form
Seed Savers Exchange
3094 North Winn Road
Decorah, IA 52101
Phone: (563) 382-5990

www.parkseed.com
Park Seed Company
3507 Cokesbury Road
Hodges, SC 29653
Phone: (800) 845-3369

www.johnnyseeds.com
Email: rstore@johnnyseeds.com
Johnny's Retail Store
Customer Fulfillment Center
955 Benton Avenue
Winslow, ME 04901
Phone: (207) 238-5327
   (Retail Store)
Phone: (877) 564-6697
   (Johnny's Seeds)

www.seedsofchange.com
Seeds of Change
P. O. Box 4908
Rancho Dominguez, CA 90220
Phone: (888) 762-7333

www.groworganic.com
Peaceful Valley Farm Supply
P. O. Box 2209
125 Clydesdale Court
Grass Valley, CA 95945
Phone: (888) 784-1722

http://organicsproutingseeds.com
Organic Sprouting Seeds
5437 W. Bavarian Pass
Minneapolis, MN 55432
Phone: (763) 502-6902

www.oikostreecrops.com
Oikos Tree Crops
P. O. Box 19425
Kalamazoo, MI 49019
Phone: (269) 624-6233

www.oldpueblocompany.com
Old Pueblo Plants &
   Seed Company
P. O. Box 86441
Tucson, AZ 85745
Phone: (866) 710-1286

www.treesofantiquity.com
Trees of Antiquity
20 Wellsona Road
Paso Robles, CA 93446
Phone: (805) 467-9909

www.raintreenursery.com
Raintree Nursery
391 Butts Road
Morton, WA 98356
Phone: (800) 391-8892

http://reneesgarden.com
Renee's Garden Seed
6060A Graham Hill
Felton, CA 95018
Phone: (831) 335-7228

www.pepperjoe.com
Pepper Joe's
3904 Kensington Court
Myrtle Beach, SC 29577
Phone: (843) 626-4507

www.richfarmgarden.com
Rich Farm Garden Supply
985 W. State Road 32
Winchester, IN 47394
Phone: (765) 584-2500

www.naturalgardening.com
Natural Gardening Company
P. O. Box 750776
Petaluma, CA 94975-0776
Phone: (707) 766-9303

www.naturescrossroads.com
Nature's Crossroads
   Earth-Friendly Seeds
230 W. Church Lane
Bloomington, IN 47403
Phone: (812) 327-9612

www.mountainvalleygrowers.com
Mountain Valley Growers, Inc.
38325 Pepperweed Road
Squaw Valley, CA 93675
Phone: (559) 338-2775

http://sprouting.com
Mumm's Sprouting Seeds, Ltd.
P. O. Box 80
Parkside, SK Canada
S0J 2A0
Phone: (306) 747-2935

www.orchardhouseheirlooms.com
Orchard House Heirlooms
216 S. Paul Street
Dowagiac, MI 49047
Phone: (269) 782-7000

www.thymegarden.com
The Thyme Garden Herb
   Company
20546M Alsea Highway
Alsea, OR 97324
Phone: (541) 487-8671

www.tomatogrowers.com
Tomato Growers
  Supply Company
P. O. Box 60015
Fort Myers, FL 33906
Phone: (888) 478-7333

http://tomatofest.com
TomatoFest Heirloom
  Tomato Seeds
Box 628
Little River, CA 95456
Phone: (707) 937-1218

www.shoptgw.com
The Gardeners Workshop Farm
P. O. Box 2987
Newport News, VA 23609
Phone: (757) 877-7159

www.livingseedcompany.com
The Living Seed Company
P. O. Box 272
San Geronimo, CA 94963
Phone: (415) 662-6855

www.tasefulgarden.com
The Tasteful Garden
973 County Road 8
Heflin, AL 36264
Phone: (256) 403-3413

http://twowingsfarm.com
Two Wings Farm Organic Seeds
4768 William Head Road
Victoria, BC Canada
V9C3Y7
Phone: (250) 478-3794

http://westwindseeds.com
Westwind Seeds & Gardenscapes,
  LLC.
6336 N. Oracle #326-246
Tucson, AZ 85704
Phone: (520) 887-2106

www.underwoodgardens.com
Underwood Gardens
P. O. Box 4995
Chino Valley, AZ 86323
Phone: (888) 878-5247

www.victoryseeds.com
Victory Seed Company
P. O. Box 192
Molalla, OR 97038
Phone: (503) 829-3126

www.thechilewoman.com
The Chile Woman
1704 S. Weimer Road
Bloomington, IN 47403
Phone: (812) 339-8321

www.seedstrust.com
Seeds Trust
P. O. Box 596
Cornville, AZ 86325
Phone: (928) 649-3315

www.selectseeds.com
Select Seeds
180 Stickney Hill Road
Union, CT 06076
Phone: (800) 684-0395

http://seeds.soggycreek.com
Soggy Creek Seed Co.
113 Chapman's Landing Road
Nipissing Village, Ontario
  P0H 1W0 Canada
Phone: (705) 724-1144

www.growitalian.com
Seeds From Italy
P. O. Box 3908
Lawrence, KS 66047
Phone: (785) 748-0959

www.southernexposure.com
Southern Exposure Seed Exchange
P. O. Box 460
Mineral, VA 23117
Phone: (540) 894-9480

www.sustainableseedco.com
Sustainable Seed Company
P. O. Box 38
Covelo, CA 95428
Phone: (707) 620-SEED

www.territorialseed.com
Territorial Seed Company
P. O. Box 158
Cottage Grove, OR 97424
Phone: (800) 626-0866

www.sowtrueseed.com
Sow True Seed
146 Church Street
Asheville, NC 28748
Phone: (828) 254-0708

www.StClareSeeds.com
St. Clare Heirloom Seeds
P. O. Box 556
Gillett, WI 54124
Email: email@stclareseeds.com

www.sunfarm.com
Sunshine Farm & Gardens
HC 67 Box 539 B
Renick, WV 24966
Phone: (304) 497-2208

www.chileplants.com
Cross Country Nurseries
P. O. Box 170
199 Kingwood-Loctown Road
Rosemont, NJ 08556-0170
Phone: (908) 996-4646

www.dixondalefarms.com
Dixondale Farms, Inc.
P. O. Box 127
Carrizo Springs, TX 78834
Phone: (877) 367-1015

www.fedcoseeds.com
Fedco Seeds
P. O. Box 520
Waterville, ME 04903
Phone: (207) 426-9900

www.mygardenofdelights.com
Garden of Delights
14560 SW 14th Street
Davie, FL 33325-4217
Phone: (954) 370-9004

www.filareefarm.com
Filaree Garlic Farm
182 Conconully Highway
Okanogan, WA 98840
Phone: (509) 422-6940

www.growincrazyacres.com
Florida Backyard Vegetable
  Gardener
5344 Culbreath Road
Brooksville, FL 34601
Phone: (352) 650-7343

www.ecogenesis.ca
Ecogenesis
General Delivery
Guelph, ON N1H 6J5
Canada
Phone: (877) 836-3693

www.eonseed.com
Eden Organic Nursery Services, Inc.
2021 SW 70th Avenue B-10
Davie, FL 33317
Phone: (954) 382-8281

www.eGardenSeed.com
eGardenSeed.com
230 Summit circle
Lafayette, CO 80026
Phone: (707) SEEDS-10

www.blueriverorgseed.com
Blue River Hybrids
27087 Timber Road
Kelly, IA 50134
Phone: (800) 370-7979

www.JLHudsonSeeds.net
J. L. Hudson, Seesman
P. O. Box 337
La Honda, CA 94020-0337
Email: inquiry@jlhudsonseeds.net

www.kitchengardensseeds.com/index
.html
John Scheepers Kitchen
    Garden Seeds
23 Tulip Drive
P. O. Box 638
Bantam, CT 06750
Phone: (860) 567-6086

www.johnnyseeds.com
Johnny's Selected Seeds
955 Benton Avenue
Winslow, ME 04901
Phone: (207) 861-3900

www.irish-eyes.com
Irish Eyes Garden Seeds
5045 Robinson Canyon Road
Ellensburg, WA 98926
Phone: (509) 964-7000

http://italianseedandtool.com
Italian Seed and Tool
HC 12 Box 510
Tatum, NM 88267
Phone: (575) 398-6111

www.justfruitsandexotics.com
Just Fruits and Exotics
30 Saint Frances St.
Crawfordville, FL 32327
Phone: (850) 926-5644

www.morgancountyseeds.com
Morgan County Seeds
18761 Kelsay Road
Barnett, MO 65011-3009
Phone: (660) 287-2400

http://kitazawaseed.com
Kitazawa Seed Company
P. O. Box 13220
Oakland, CA 94661-3220
Phone: (510) 595-1188

www.alseed.com
Albert Lea Seed House
1414 West Main
P. O. Box 127
Albert Lea, MN 56007
Phone: (800) 352-5247

www.2bseeds.com
2BSEEDS, LLC.
5023 W 120th Avenue #312
Broomfield, CO 80020
Phone: (800) 833-5988

http://afewgoodplants.com
A Few Good Plants
7595 S. W. Highway DD
El Dorado Springs, MO 64744
Phone: (417) 876-7139

www.annieheirloomseeds.com
Annie's Heirloom Seeds
12123 Darby Road
Clarksville, MI 48815
Phone: (800) 313-9140

www.botanicalinterests.com
Botanical Interests
660 Compton Street
Broomfield, CO 80020
Phone: (720) 880-7293

http://rareseeds.com
Baker Creek Heirloom
  Seed Company
2278 Baker Creek Road
Mansfield, MO 65704
Phone: (417) 924-8917

http://marysheirloomseeds.com
Mary's Heirloom Seeds
1850 Monroe Street
Hollywood, FL 33020
Phone: (954) 364-8841

www.centuryfarmorchards.com
Century Farm Orchards
1614 Rice Road
Reidsville, NC 27320
Phone: (336) 349-5709

www.american-organic.com
American Hybrids and Organic
  Seed Company
P. O. Box 385
Warren, IL 61087
Phone: (855) 945-2449

Box Garden Organics
2740 Central Avenue
Ammon, ID 83406-7760
Phone: (208) 227-3282

www.bighorsecreekfarm.com
P. O. Box 70
Lansing, NC 28643
Phone: (336) 384-1134

www.oldvaapples.com
Urban Homestead
818 Cumberland Street
Bristol, VA 24201
Phone: (276) 466-2931

www.thetreecenter.com
The Tree Center
123 Gov. Bridge Road
Davidsonville, MD 21035
Phone: (888) 476-0123

www.skyfiregardenseeds.com
Skyfire Garden Seed Company
100 S. College Avenue
Salina, KS 67401
Phone: (785) 577-1979

www.jungseed.com
Jung Seed Company
335 S. High Street
Randolph, WI 53957
Phone: (920) 326-3121

www.alcasoft.com/bostonmountain
Boston Mountain Nurseries
20189 N Highway 71
Mountainburg, AR 72946
Phone: (479) 369-2007

www.eternalseed.ca
Eternal Seed
2309 Zilinsky Road - Kelly Creek
Powell River, BC Canada
V8A 5C1
Phone: (604) 487-1304

www.buylandscapingplants.com
Indian Creek Nursery
156 Main Street
Altamont, TN 37301
Phone: (931) 692-4837

www.seed-bank.ca
Seed Bank
108 Bruton Street
Port Hope, ON L1A 1V3
Canada

www.natureandnurtureseeds.com
Nature and Nurture Seeds
114 8th Street
Ann Arbor, MI 48103
Phone: (734) 929-0802

www.johnsonnursery.com
Johnson Nursery, Inc.
1352 Big Creek Road
Ellijay, GA 30536
Phone: (888) 276-3187

www.paireroadorganic.com
Prairie Road Organic Seed
9824 79th Street SE
Fullerton, ND 58441
Phone: (701) 883-4416

www.sagethymes.com
Sage Thymes
8550 W Ohio Place
Lakewood, CO 80226
Phone: (720) 480-1017

http://PeaceSeedsLive.blogspot.com
Peace Seeds
2385 SE Thompson Street
Corvallis, OR 97333-1919
Phone: (541) 752-0421

Metric Conversion Charts

1 teaspoon = 5 ml
1 dessertspoon = 10 ml
1/2 fluid ounce = 3 teaspoons = 1 tablespoon = 15 ml
1 fluid ounce = 2 tablespoons = 1/8 cup = 30 ml
2 fluid ounces = 4 tablespoons = 1/4 cup = 60 ml
4 fluid ounces = 8 tablespoons = 1/2 cup = 120 ml
8 fluid ounces = 16 tablespoons = 1 cup = 235 ml
16 fluid ounces = 1 pint = 1/2 quart = 2 cups = 475 ml
128 fluid ounces = 8 pints = 4 quarts = 1 gallon = 1L

1 gram = 0.035 ounces
1 ounce = 28.35 grams
1 kg = 35 ounces / 2.2 lbs.
Converter for U.S., British, Europe, and Australia:
    www.convert-me.com/en/convert/cooking/

Oven Temperatures:

Gas	Fahrenheit	Celsius	Temp.
1/2	250	120	Very slow
1	275	140	
2	300	150	Slow
3	325	170	
4	350	180	Moderate
5	375	190	
6	400	200	Mod. Hot
7	425	220	
8	450	230	Hot
9	475	240	Very Hot

Grams	Ounces	Grams	Ounces/Pounds	Kilograms	Ounces/Pounds
10	1/4	350	12	1kg	2 1/4 lbs.
15	1/2	375	13	1.25kg	2 lbs. 12 oz.
25	1	400	14	1.5kg	3 lbs. 5 oz.
50	1 3/4	425	15	2kg	4 1/2 lbs.
75	2 3/4	450	1 lb.	2.25kg	5 lbs.
100	3 1/2	500	1 lb. 2 oz.	2.5kg	5 1/2 lbs.
150	5 1/2	700	1 1/2 lb.	3kg	6 1/2 lbs.
175	6	750	1 lb. 10 oz.		
200	7				
225	8				
250	9				
275	9 3/4				
300	10 1/2				

www.ingramcontent.com/pod-product-compliance
Lightning Source LLC
Chambersburg PA
CBHW070834310526
45788CB00017B/931